# Mobility, Sexuality and AIDS

Over the past two decades, population mobility has intensified and become more diverse, raising important questions concerning the health and well-being of people who are mobile as well as communities of origin and destination.

Ongoing concerns have been voiced about possible links between mobility and HIV, with calls being made to contain or control migrant populations, and debate linking HIV with issues of global security and surveillance being fuelled. This volume challenges common assumptions about mobility, HIV and AIDS. A series of interlinked chapters prepared by international experts explores the experiences of people who are mobile as they relate to sexuality and to HIV susceptibility and impact. The various chapters discuss the factors that contribute to the vulnerability of different mobile groups but also examine the ways in which agency, resilience and adaptation shape lived experience and help people protect themselves throughout the mobility process. Looking at diverse forms of migration and mobility – covering flight from conflict, poverty and exploitation, through labour migration to 'sex tourism' – the book reports on research findings from around the world, including the USA, the UK, sub-Saharan Africa, Australia, Central America and China.

*Mobility, Sexuality and AIDS* recognises the complex relationships between individual circumstances, population mobility and community and state response. It is invaluable reading for policy makers, students and practitioners working in the fields of migration, development studies, anthropology, sociology, geography and public health.

**Felicity Thomas** is a Research Fellow at the Thomas Coram Research Unit, Institute of Education, University of London. Active in the field of international development for over ten years, she has been involved in a number of research and action-based projects with refugees and asylum seekers living in sub-Saharan Africa and in the UK. Her research interests focus on the socio-economic and emotional impacts of HIV and AIDS, migrant health and well-being, and HIV treatment seeking and management.

**Mary Haour-Knipe** has worked in the field of migration and HIV since 1989, leading a European Union working group assessing HIV prevention activities for migrants and travellers in Europe, evaluating HIV prevention programmes amongst migrant communities, and working as senior advisor on migration and HIV/AIDS, then on migration and health, at the International Organization for Migration. She has also served as an advisor on HIV-related migration issues for the Joint United Nations Programme on HIV/AIDS.

**Peter Aggleton** is Professor of Education in the Thomas Coram Research Unit, Institute of Education, University of London and Visiting Professor at the University of Oslo and the University of New South Wales. He is the author and editor of over thirty books and internationally renowned for his work on sexuality and HIV. He is editor of the journal *Culture, Health and Sexuality*, senior editor of *Global Public Health* and associate editor of *Health Education Research* and *AIDS Education and Prevention*.

# Sexuality, Culture and Health series

Edited by
Peter Aggleton
*Institute of Education, University of London, UK*
Richard Parker
*Columbia University, New York, USA*
Sonia Corrêa
*ABIA, Rio de Janeiro, Brazil*
Gary Dowsett
*La Trobe University, Melbourne, Australia*
Shirley Lindenbaum
*City University of New York, USA*

This new series of books offers cutting-edge analysis, current theoretical perspectives and up-to-the-minute ideas concerning the interface between sexuality, public health, human rights, culture and social development. It adopts a global and interdisciplinary perspective in which the needs of poorer countries are given equal status to those of richer nations. The books are written with a broad range of readers in mind, and will be invaluable to students, academics and those working in policy and practice. The series also aims to serve as a spur to practical action in an increasingly globalised world.

Available in the series:

**Culture, Society and Sexuality**
A reader, 2nd ed.
*Edited by Peter Aggleton and Richard Parker*

**Dying to be Men**
Youth, masculinity and social exclusion
*Gary T. Barker*

**Sex, Drugs and Young People**
International perspectives
*Edited by Peter Aggleton, Andrew Ball and Purnima Mane*

**Promoting Young People's Sexual Health**
International perspectives
*Edited by Roger Ingham and Peter Aggleton*

**Sexuality, Health and Human Rights**
*Sonia Corrêa, Rosalind Petchesky and Richard Parker*

**Mobility, Sexuality and AIDS**
*Edited by Felicity Thomas, Mary Haour-Knipe and Peter Aggleton*

# Mobility, Sexuality and AIDS

Edited by Felicity Thomas,
Mary Haour-Knipe and Peter Aggleton

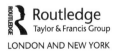

Routledge
Taylor & Francis Group

LONDON AND NEW YORK

First published 2010
by Routledge
2 Park Square, Milton Park, Abingdon, Oxon, OX14 4RN

Simultaneously published in the USA and Canada
by Routledge
711 Third Avenue, New York, NY 10017, USA

*Routledge is an imprint of the Taylor & Francis Group, an informa business*

Typeset in Baskerville by
Taylor & Francis Books

*British Library Cataloguing in Publication Data*
A catalogue record for this book is available from the British Library

*Library of Congress Cataloguing in Publication Data*
Mobility, sexuality, and AIDS / edited by Felicity Thomas, Mary Haour-Knipe,
and Peter Aggleton.
    p. ; cm
    Includes bibliographical references.
    1. AIDS (Disease)–Epidemiology 2. Emigration and immigration–Health
aspects. 3. Medical geography. I. Thomas, Felicity. II. Haour-Knipe, Mary.
III. Aggleton, Peter.
    [DNLM: 1. HIV Infections–transmission. 2. Emigration and Immigration.
3. Risk Assessment. 4. Sexual Behavior. 5. Socioeconomic Factors.
WC 503.3 M687 2009]
    RA643.8.M63 2009
    362.196'9792–dc22                                         2009014389

ISBN10: 0-415-47777-8 (hbk)
ISBN10: 0-203-86914-1 (ebk)

ISBN13: 978-0-415-47777-2 (hbk)
ISBN13: 978-0-203-86914-7 (ebk)

# Contents

## Mobility and pleasure

## Mobility and work

# Figures

# Tables

# Contributors

**Jane Anderson** (Homerton University Hospital NHS Foundation Trust and Barts and the London School of Medicine and Dentistry, UK) is a consultant physician in HIV Medicine and Director of the Centre for the Study of Sexual Health and HIV. Research exploring relationships between the biological and psychosocial aspects of HIV infection is embedded in the clinical setting and reflects the diversity of the patient population in East London. HIV in minority ethnic and migrant populations in the UK, many of whom are women, is at the centre of the research programme.

**Islene Araujo de Carvalho** holds a PhD in medicine and diplomas in gynaecology, community health and international health. She has worked in government and non-government organizations in Brazil and other Latin American countries, East Timor and several African countries. While based in Zimbabwe she implemented and managed health programming for the International Organization for Migration, focusing especially on integrating HIV prevention activities within humanitarian emergencies. She later managed IOM's worldwide health and HIV programming for mobile populations and migrants. She is currently a technical officer for the department of gender, women and health of the World Health Organization, focusing on the intersection between HIV and gender.

**Ousman Bah** is a Gambian ethnographer with seven years of anthropological research experience, specifically relating to the interaction between local cultures, health-seeking behaviour, and national policies. Based at the Medical Research Council Laboratories' field station in Farafenni, he studied rural communities' perceptions, attitudes and behaviours regarding both malaria and HIV/AIDS. More recently, he has been interested in the study of sexualities within tourism, specifically focusing on the place of gender, generation, race and religiosity. His recent publications have appeared in the journals *Culture, Health and Sexuality*, *Qualitative Research* and the *African Journal of Reproductive Health*.

**Lorraine van Blerk** currently works as a Lecturer in Human Geography at the University of Reading, UK. Her research expertise focuses on the lives of young people in situations of poverty across east and southern Africa including street children, young commercial sex workers and children affected by AIDS. She is also particularly interested in exploring new ways of undertaking participatory and ethical research with young people.

**Héctor Carrillo** is Associate Professor of Sociology and Gender Studies at Northwestern University, USA. He is the author of *The Night is Young: Sexuality in Mexico in the Time of AIDS* (University of Chicago Press, 2002) which received the Ruth Benedict Prize from the American Anthropological Association. His current research focuses on the sexuality and HIV risk of Mexican immigrants living in the USA. In collaboration with researchers in Mexico, he is also investigating the cultural meanings of adult male circumcision – which some support as an HIV prevention measure – among Mexican immigrants.

In over 15 years of professional work in HIV prevention, **H. Daniel Castellanos** has participated in a broad range of programmatic activities and research projects concerning social and behavioural interventions. A lesbian, gay, bisexual and transgender (LGBT) activist and a graduate of the Mailman School of Public Health at Columbia University, USA, he has conducted research on male sex work and LGBT youth activism in the Dominican Republic, health access barriers and facilitators among LGBT immigrants in New York City and homelessness among young gay men in New York City. He is particularly interested in the health opportunities and challenges of increased LGBT global activism and domestic and international migration of young gay men.

**Karl L. Dehne** is the Senior Advisor, Health Systems and Multisectoral Responses in UNAIDS, Geneva. Karl has worked on AIDS prevention and care for 25 years, including in UNAIDS as Team Leader, Eastern Europe; Team Leader, Security and Humanitarian Response; Senior Advisor on HIV and Drug Use; and Country Coordinator, Zimbabwe. In the World Health Organization he worked as Medical Officer and Epidemiologist. From 1998 to 2000 Karl was a Lecturer at the University of Heidelberg, Germany, where he led the UNAIDS Collaborating Centre on AIDS Strategic Planning and Operational Research in Eastern Europe. He also was District Medical Officer in Zimbabwe and Health Project Coordinator in Burkina Faso. Karl holds an MD (University of Heidelberg, Germany), a PhD in Population Geography and an MPH (both University of Leeds, UK).

**Chenoa A. Flippen** is an Assistant Professor of Sociology at the University of Pennsylvania, USA. Her primary research interests relate to racial and ethnic stratification, including such diverse topics as minority ageing, inequality in wealth accumulation, and the impact of residential segregation on minority home ownership and housing appreciation. Her contribution to this volume relates to work on Hispanic immigrant adaptation in Durham, North

Carolina. This project examines the impact of migration on gender roles and health behaviours, as well as the labour market experiences of undocumented migrants and the role of income pooling in surviving low-wage work. The common theme uniting these endeavours, which combine both quantitative and qualitative methodologies, is an interest in how structural conditions affect minorities' life chances.

**Jennifer S. Hirsch** is Associate Professor of Sociomedical Sciences in the Mailman School of Public Health at Columbia University, USA. Her research interests include the comparative anthropology of love, gender and sexuality, US–Mexico migration, and HIV. She is the author of *A Courtship after Marriage: Sexuality and Love in Mexican Transnational Families* (University of California Press, 2003) and co-author (with Daniel Jordan Smith, Holly Wardlow, Harriet Phinney, Shanti Parikh and Constance Nathanson) of *The Secret: Love, Marriage, and HIV.*

**Mark Hunter** is Assistant Professor of Geography at the University of Toronto, Canada. He is a graduate of the University of Sussex, UK; the University of KwaZulu-Natal, South Africa; and the University of California at Berkeley, USA, where he completed his PhD. Since 2000 he has been researching AIDS in the KwaZulu-Natal province of South Africa, combining political economy and ethnographic methods. A book manuscript resulting from this project is currently under review. He has published articles in journals that include *African Studies, Social Science & Medicine, Transformation,* and *Culture, Health and Sexuality.*

**Henrike Körner**'s background is in systemic functional linguistics. She worked in English language and literacy education and is currently a Senior Research Fellow at the National Centre in HIV Social Research at the University of New South Wales in Sydney, Australia. Her research focuses on gay men's discourses of 'risk' in the context of HIV infection, doctor/patient interactions, HIV/AIDS as it affects people from culturally and linguistically diverse backgrounds, representation of HIV and hepatitis C-related issues in the medical and popular media. Her most recent work is concerned with general practitioners diagnosing depression in gay men, and discourses of depression.

**Sergio Meneses Navarro** holds an MD and MA, and has a PhD in Public Health. He is currently working as Chief of the Department of Health Systems Research at the Regional Center of Research in Public Health, Tapachula, Chiapas, Mexico.

**Stella Nyanzi** is a medical anthropologist with the Law, Gender and Sexuality Research Project in the Faculty of Law at Makerere University. She has 12 years of social science research experience on diverse social-cultural phenomena relating to HIV/AIDS. She has published on sexual behaviours of diverse sub-cultures in Uganda and The Gambia including school pupils, rural youths, pregnant mothers, people living with HIV/AIDS, commercial sex workers, motorbike taxi riders, beach boys, widows and widowers. She is also interested in investigating alternative medicines, faith healing and health policy. Her most recent book is *How to be a 'Proper' Woman in the Time of AIDS* (Nordic Africa Institute, 2007, with Katja Jassey).

**Kennedy Nyabuti Ondimu** PhD is currently Associate Professor of Geography and Dean, Faculty of Environmental Studies and Resources Development, Egerton University, Kenya. His areas of research interests include population dynamics and health outcomes, health impact assessment, gender issues in health, and population growth and natural resource management in Kenya.

**Mark B. Padilla** is Assistant Professor in the Department of Health Behavior and Health Education and Adjunct Assistant Professor in the Department of Anthropology at the University of Michigan, USA. He is a medical anthropologist with cross-training in public health, and has worked for 10 years on HIV/AIDS research and interventions in Latin America and the Caribbean. His books include *Caribbean Pleasure Industry: Tourism, Sexuality and AIDS in the Dominican Republic* (University of Chicago Press, 2007), which won the 2008 Ruth Benedict Prize from the American Anthropological Association, and *Love and Globalization: Transformations of Intimacy in the Contemporary World* (Vanderbilt University Press, 2007). The primary focus of his ethnographic research is the intersection of gender, sexuality, and HIV/AIDS among vulnerable populations in Latin America and the Caribbean. He is currently conducting a project funded by the National Institute on Alcohol Abuse and Alcoholism on the intersection of alcohol consumption and HIV risk in Dominican tourism areas.

**Emilio A. Parrado** is an Associate Professor in the Department of Sociology at the University of Pennsylvania, USA. His research focuses on issues of immigration and immigrant adaptation, especially among Latinos in the USA. He is currently the principal investigator of the project 'Gender, migration, and HIV risks among Hispanics: a tri-national design'. The main objective of the project is to understand the connection between migration, gender relations and HIV risks among Mexican and Honduran migrants to Durham, North Carolina. The research design combines quantitative and qualitative methodologies. Results from this project are presented in this volume.

**Preeti Patel** is a Lecturer in Military Sociology in the Department of War Studies and the King's Centre for Military Health Research at King's College London, UK. Prior to joining King's College London, she worked as a Lecturer in Global Health at the London School of Hygiene & Tropical Medicine, UK. Her research interests are in the politics of health and security in fragile states, international peacekeeping, civil-military relations, conflict and development, governance and transnational corporations, sexual violence, gender and HIV/AIDS.

**Bayard Roberts** has worked in the Conflict and Health Programme at the London School of Hygiene & Tropical Medicine, UK, since 2005. His research and publications cover a variety of topics including the delivery of reproductive health services in conflict-affected countries, validating a new method to estimate mortality in conflict-affected populations and researching determinants of health of conflict-affected populations in northern Uganda and Southern Sudan. Bayard previously spent four years working with reproductive health and HIV/AIDS programmes in Afghanistan, Pakistan, Uganda and elsewhere, and he has also conducted consultancy work on forced migration and health.

**Jacobo Schifter** teaches on the history of sexual rights and on gender and human rights at the United Nations' University of Peace, as well as on gen-ocide at the University of Costa Rica and at the University for International Cooperation. Jacobo has authored a number of books on health and sex-ualities, his two most recent being *Terminal*, a study of breast cancer and its treatments in Costa Rica, and *15 Minutes of Fame*, a historical novel on being gay and Jewish in Costa Rica and in the USA in the 1960s. His most recent research is focused on intolerance and anti-Semitism in the Central America region.

**Daniel Jordan Smith** is Associate Professor of Anthropology and Associate Director of the Population Studies and Training Center at Brown University, USA. He has conducted research on HIV/AIDS in Nigeria since the 1990s and has published widely on this topic in journals such as *AIDS, American Journal of Public Health, Culture, Health and Sexuality, Medical Anthropology* and *Studies in Family Planning*. His book *A Culture of Corruption: Everyday Deception and Popular Discontent in Nigeria* (Princeton University Press, 2007) won the 2008 Margaret Mead Award. He is also co-author (with Jennifer S. Hirsch, Holly Wardlow, Harriet Phinney, Shanti Parikh and Constance Nathanson) of a forthcoming book, *The Secret: Love, Marriage, and HIV* (Vanderbilt University Press).

**Leonardo Uribe** received his PhD in Public Health from the University of North Carolina at Chapel Hill, USA and was a postdoctoral research associ-ate at the Social Science Research Institute of Duke University, USA. He is currently a researcher and health promoter in his native Colombia. His work centres on the public health aspects of Hispanic immigration to the USA. He has worked extensively with the Hispanic community in Durham, North Carolina. His dissertation investigated issues of social support, social isolation, and neighbourhood conditions and how they relate to sexual risk behaviours, alcohol abuse and depression among recent migrants.

**Holly Wardlow** is an Associate Professor of Anthropology at the University of Toronto, where she teaches classes in gender, medical anthropology and global health. She is the author of *Wayward Women: Sexuality and Agency in a New Guinea Society* (University of California Press, 2006), an ethnography about 'passenger women', a common local term for female sex workers. She has also co-edited two books, *The Making of Global and Local Modernities in Melanesia: Humiliation, Transformation and the Nature of Cultural Change* (co-editor, Joel Robbins) and *Modern Loves: The Anthropology of Romantic Courtship and Companionate Marriage* (co-editor, Jennifer S. Hirsch).

**Xiushi Yang** is a social demographer and Professor in the Department of Sociology and Criminal Justice at the Old Dominion University, USA. For the past 15 years, his research has focused on the impact of migration and socioeconomic changes on reproductive and HIV risk behaviours in China. He is currently the principal investigator of a United States National Institute of Child Health and Human Development-funded behavioural intervention to reduce HIV risk of sexual and drug use behaviours among female entertainment workers in Shanghai. He has published extensively in the field.

# Acknowledgements

We would like to thank Daisy Ellis for assisting in the production of this book. Special thanks are also due to the authors and publishers who gave permission to reprint various excerpts and illustrations from some of the chapters collected here:

- Google Maps, for permission to reprint aerial photograph of *La Maldita Vecindad* (Figure 3.2).
- Elsevier Limited, for permission to reprint data displayed in Table 7.1.
- University Press of America, for permission to reprint excerpts from Schifter, J. (2005) 'Mongers in heaven'.
- Elsevier Limited, for permission to reprint excerpts from Hunter, M. (2007) 'The changing political economy of sex in South Africa: the significance of unemployment and inequalities to the scale of the AIDS pandemic', *Social Science & Medicine*, 64(3).
- Organization for Social Science Research in Eastern and Southern Africa (OSSREA), for permission to reprint data displayed in Tables 12.1, 12.2 and 12.3.
- Pion Limited, London, for permission to reprint excerpts from Yang, X. (2006) 'Temporary migration and HIV risk behaviors in China', *Environment and Planning A*, 38(8).

# Abbreviations

| | |
|---|---|
| AIDS | Acquired immune deficiency syndrome |
| ALAFA | Apparel Lesotho Alliance to Fight AIDS |
| CBPR | Community Based Participatory Research |
| HIV | Human immunodeficiency virus |
| HSRC | Human Science Research Council |
| IAWG | Interagency Working Group |
| IDP | Internally displaced person |
| ILO | International Labour Organization |
| KAPB | Knowledge, Attitudes, Practices and Beliefs |
| LGBT | Lesbian, gay, bisexual, transgender |
| LGBTQ | Lesbian, gay, bisexual, transgender and queer |
| MHAHS | Multicultural HIV/AIDS and Hepatitis C Service |
| NHS | National Health Service |
| NSRRT | National Sex and Reproduction Research Team |
| PSU | Primary sampling unit |
| RNA | Ribonucleic acid |
| STI | Sexually transmitted infection |
| UN | United Nations |
| UNAIDS | United Nations Programme on HIV/AIDS |
| UNFPA | United Nations Population Fund |
| UNGASS | United Nations General Assembly Special Session |
| UNHCR | United Nations High Commissioner for Refugees |
| UNIFEM | United Nations Development Fund for Women |
| UNOCHA | United Nations Office for the Coordination of Humanitarian Affairs |
| VCT | Voluntary counselling and testing |
| WHO | World Health Organization |

# Introduction

## Mobility, sexuality and AIDS

*Felicity Thomas, Mary Haour-Knipe and
Peter Aggleton*

Over the past two decades, processes of globalization have radically altered the intensity, scale, pace and diversity of global connections. The movement of individuals and groups has in turn been facilitated by the growth of global communication and transportation, as well as by the existence of social networks and groups of people who have already migrated, and who can help family members and friends settle into a new society. While globalization has strengthened economic links across regions, changing demographics, inequalities of opportunity, conflict and unrest, changes in sociocultural norms and expectations, and the pursuit of individual desire and aspiration have also – in varying ways – intensified the tendencies for people to move across and within regions, nations and localities.

As population movement becomes more complex, concerns have been voiced about potential links between mobility, health and wellbeing in general, and about the possibility of transmission of infectious diseases in particular. Since it creates a bridge between regions and peoples that had been socially and spatially isolated, population mobility has long been linked to disease outbreaks and epidemics (Kraut 1995; Apostolopoulos and Sonmez 2007; Jatrana *et al.* 2007). This historical concern about mobility and infectious diseases became particularly apparent in recent times with widespread fears – at least in the early years of the epidemic – about the transmission of HIV. In the 1980s and early 1990s the global imagination surrounding AIDS was fed by a plethora of fear-producing images (Patton 2002). Such fears also influenced a popularly perceived need to in some way contain or control various migrant populations (Coker 2003), and have also played a role in fuelling debates linking HIV with issues of global security and surveillance (Prins 2004; Ingram 2005).

Certainly influenced by such fears, or more specifically by concerns regarding the nourishing of such fears and of stigmatising mobile populations, much of the initial published literature on migration and HIV was very prudent. Relatively little was published, and, along with much of the research concerning HIV and AIDS at the time, what did appear remained largely epidemiological and behavioural in nature. By the mid-1990s, however, and within HIV and AIDS research, the limitations of behaviouralist approaches to understanding the transmission of the virus were becoming evident, leading to increased academic and policy-based recognition that HIV and AIDS were not solely medical issues but were best understood through a broad 'biosocial' lens (Farmer 1999). This more socially oriented focus allowed the epidemic to be considered in relation to wider economic and cultural processes, and within the broader structures and meanings that shape sexual experience in different contexts and settings (Herdt 1997; Parker *et al.* 2000; Parker 2001; Manalansan 2006).

Following the same trends, much of the literature on HIV and migration since that time has thus focused on the specific HIV-related risks and vulnerabilities experienced by mobile populations, the communities that host them, and the communities to which they return. Those involved in labour migration have received particular attention, especially men who move from developing areas in search of improved livelihood opportunities in other regions, countries or continents (see, for example, Campbell 1997; Lurie *et al.* 2003). More recently, however, the scope of interest has widened to examine 'mobile' populations, thus taking into account the increasingly wide array of situations, circumstances and time scales within which people from a diverse variety of countries and backgrounds move from place to place. Key populations include, amongst others, migrant labourers, refugees, internally displaced people, sex workers, tourists, professionals and people returning 'home'. In addition, increasing attention has been paid not only to the diversity of the ways in which globalisation processes bring these groups into contact with host and home communities, but also to the ways in which they may interact with one other.

Largely as a result of the HIV pandemic, recognition of the more holistic contexts and processes which shape sexual experience, and the emergence of intellectual interest in feminism, ethnic studies and lesbian, gay, bisexual, transgender and queer studies, the past two decades have seen a parallel surge in the development of academic work on human sexuality (Kimmel and Plante 2004; Parker and Aggleton 2007). Importantly, however, it is really only in the past decade that the study of sexuality in the context of transnational and global mobility has intensified, with literature now appearing in the fields of anthropology, sociology, geography, history, and public health. Two key lines of enquiry have developed as these relate to HIV and AIDS. The first looks at the ways in which mobility can influence self-perceptions and actions as people move, and find themselves exposed to what Herdt (1997:3) describes as new 'cultures of sexuality'. Secondly, more recent literature has begun to recognize that far from homogenizing ideas about sexuality, processes of globalization have often hybridized sexual ideologies, behaviours and identities. It is increasingly recognized that many of the categories, conceptions and models used in a Western context to describe these ideologies, behaviours and identities can neither be applied universally, nor considered static (Parker 2001; Manalansan 2006).

Despite this more 'insider' approach to understanding sexuality, the nature and legacy of the HIV pandemic have overwhelmingly been to problematize sexual experience, particularly in research related to sexuality and health. As many of the chapters in this book argue, understanding the various risks and vulnerabilities faced by some mobile populations with regards to HIV and AIDS – as well as those of host and home communities – remains a key concern for HIV-based policy, programming and intervention which cannot, and must not, be ignored. However increased recognition of the social and cultural construction of sexuality – and of the various ways in which HIV and the social spaces created by population movement can themselves be conceptualized and experienced – raises important questions with respect to the risk and vulnerability faced by people who are mobile, and by those with whom they interact.

Recognition that the ways in which a person's sexuality – or the ways his or her sexuality is perceived by others – can influence his or her situation, has taken place in parallel with wider trends within the social sciences which stress the importance of actor agency, adaptation and resilience for understanding the fluidity and diversity of lived experience. *Mobility, Sexuality and AIDS* attempts to consolidate some of the key developments which have emerged across the social sciences which bring together this array of issues in their examination of the interface between mobile individuals and populations, sexuality, HIV and AIDS. The volume emerged from the editors' sense of the potential importance of such insights for those working at the intersections of mobility and health, either as practitioners or as academics. We felt that this new book could help increase understanding of the complex inter-linkages between these new insights, and deepen knowledge of the heterogeneous priorities, needs, actions and experiences of different mobile populations, and of the home and host communities with whom they liaise.

We have tried to organize the book in a way that will provide insight as to how mobility, sexuality, HIV and AIDS intersect within the wider social, political, economic and cultural structures and processes that take place at different scales: from the micro level of the family and household to the macro levels of health-related policy making. In so doing, we have organized not by geographical region or by migration trajectory, but have identified three over-arching themes which recur in the chapters that make up the volume: mobility and the experience of the self, mobility and pleasure, and mobility and work. Particular issues – such as increasing mobility of women, the need to examine the interconnections between structure and agency, the potential importance of the church, or the unintended consequences of seemingly benevolent labour migration policies – appear in a number of the chapters. Similarly, movement between certain geographical areas where research on mobility, sexuality and HIV has been particularly strong, such as Central America and the USA, or between various countries in Africa, is discussed in several different sections.

Chapter 1 sets the context by providing an important overview of epidemiological studies of HIV prevalence amongst international migrants compared with the populations of destination countries. While it has frequently been hypothesized that the HIV-related risks that result from mobility increase migrants' exposure to HIV and increase the likelihood of its transmission, Islene Araujo de

Carvalho, Mary Haour-Knipe and Karl L. Dehne stress the often overlooked fact that relatively little rigorous evidence exists to support such claims. What studies are available are often based on small sample sizes, tend to focus on migrants from areas with generalised HIV epidemics, and over-represent migrants from groups considered to be at heightened risk of HIV transmission. The authors call for the creation of more solid evidence on which to base important policy formulation, and for more nuanced accounts concerning links between mobility, sexuality and HIV.

## Mobility and the experience of the self

The section on mobility and the experience of the self brings together five chapters that examine some of the crucial factors structuring decision-making amongst people who are mobile, their experiences as they relate to identity and selfhood, and the ways in which these intersect with sexuality and with HIV transmission and impact. These issues are developed in depth by Héctor Carrillo (Chapter 2), who focuses on Mexican men's migration to the USA. Carrillo examines the ways in which sexuality and sexual identity can drive migration, as they enable the pursuit of sexual practices and identities that many men feel would be constrained in Mexico. Acknowledging that mobility and migration are rarely a matter of individual decision alone, Carrillo explores the ways in which sexual motivations for migration intertwine with cultural and familial expectations and norms. Of particular concern here is the perceived need of men who identify themselves as gay or bisexual to avoid the possible negative repercussions for their families in Mexico that might arise if their sexual identity and practices become publicly known, and the challenges this can pose for them in terms of HIV and sexual health.

Taking a broader perspective and examining the ways that wider structural processes can influence HIV risk, Emilio A. Parrado, Chenoa A. Flippen and Leonardo Uribe (Chapter 3) next examine the ways in which particular neighbourhood contexts can concentrate certain disadvantages, and also create pressures amongst Latino male migrants in the USA to engage in unprotected sex with casual partners and sex workers. They not only emphasise the structural disadvantages that inhibit the formation of protective interpersonal relationships, but also draw important conclusions about the need for policy makers to develop family-based migration policies. In the following chapter, Bayard Roberts and Preeti Patel (Chapter 4) examine evidence concerning the links between conflict, forced migration and the spread of HIV. Drawing upon evidence from across sub-Saharan Africa, they make useful observations on the heterogeneity of refugees and internally displaced peoples, arguing that the complexity of conflict situations may increase some people's vulnerability to HIV in certain circumstances, but may also act as a protective factor in other situations. Roberts and Patel explain that the difficulties of gaining reliable research results can lead to misinformed and ineffective programming that runs the risk of stigmatising displaced persons as carriers of disease, and make a convincing case that new approaches must be developed for rigorous and in-depth research at the interface between conflict, forced migration and HIV.

The penultimate chapters of this section turn to the impact of HIV and AIDS, looking at migrants' interactions with health and support services. Henrike Körner (Chapter 5) focuses on the various ways sexual identity and ideas about individualist and collectivist health-seeking behaviours can influence the ability of HIV-positive migrants from Asia, Latin America and southern Europe to access support services in Australia. Körner argues that services to promote migrant health and wellbeing need to be informed by far greater understanding of the ways people from different cultures and backgrounds perceive their health, their sexuality and their self in relation to others, in their immediate community and beyond. In the following chapter (Chapter 6) Jane Anderson takes many of these same issues further, with a detailed examination of the constraints facing HIV-positive African migrants accessing treatment and care in the UK, and the ways in which gender, sexual identity and sexual lifestyles can influence emotional wellbeing and lived experience. She concludes by calling for further research on the ways that HIV itself can impact on a person's ability to pursue and enact their sexuality, and argues that greater understanding of such issues would raise the probability that the most appropriate treatment and care are provided.

## Mobility and pleasure

The chapters in the 'Mobility and pleasure' section explore the various ways in which the pursuit of pleasure and an enhanced sense of wellbeing can act as key catalysts for population movement. While several of the chapters in this section focus on the pleasures sought by tourists seeking sexual relations in foreign countries, they also discuss the motivations and experiences of those providing such experiences, and the ways they, too, make decisions to fulfil particular outcomes and aspirations. In so doing, the chapters in this section examine the often complex and seemingly contradictory concepts of agency and exploitation, and the ways in which these intersect with sexual experience and HIV risk and vulnerability. This is well illustrated in the chapter by Mark B. Padilla and H. Daniel Castellanos (Chapter 7) who explore the ways in which particular social spaces provided by tourism in the Dominican Republic come to stand in for the global experiences desired by – but unobtainable to – many local children and young men. Whilst this enables opportunities for sexual experience and expression beyond the normative constraints of local life, the authors explain that engaging with the 'global' via sexual relations with tourists raises important questions in the community about the longer-term influences of such actions on 'local' experiences of personhood, behaviour, and moral integrity and impacts upon the ways that people map and respond to their perceptions of HIV risk across different social environments.

Stella Nyanzi and Ousman Bah (Chapter 8) continue along similar lines, providing detailed insight into the motivations of *bumsters* – beach boys in The Gambia – in their pursuit of relationships with (often older) Western women tourists. Challenging conventional notions which position tourists as the exploiters, and also refuting official discourse in which *bumsters* are represented as uneducated and opportunistic delinquents, Nyanzi and Bah explore the creative strategies *bumsters* employ to foster relationships with Western women in the hope that such alliances may bring economic gain, and ultimately enable them to migrate to the West. Whilst this may enable young Gambian men to fulfil the sociocultural expectations placed upon them to provide for family members, it also allows them to exert a form of masculine sexuality beyond that which is deemed acceptable in day-to-day Gambian life, and at the same time opens up the potential for unprotected sex with multiple partners. This theme is developed further in Jacobo Schifter and Felicity Thomas's chapter (Chapter 9) which examines the frequency and ease with which American and European men can travel to Costa Rica to escape the drudgeries of home life and to fulfil their sexual desires and fantasies with young women sex workers. Drawing upon data collected via internet chat rooms, Schifter and Thomas offer a unique insight into the ways in which men pursue these 'fantasy' relationships, and also how the medium of the internet helps them share and legitimise their experiences, and foster a collective attitude of denial regarding the risks of HIV transmission. As with the previous chapter, Schifter and Thomas focus attention on the complexity of factors influencing the lives and actions of the sex workers, exploring the ways in which their relatively harsh economic circumstances intertwine with their individual aspirations to improve their socioeconomic standing and live more comfortable lives.

In the following chapter (Chapter 10), Jennifer S. Hirsch and Sergio Meneses Navarro use ethnographic data from several of their own studies to develop a subtle examination of the ways in which Mexican men express their sexuality during annual visits home to their families. In this discussion, they explore the ways in which the men's enhanced social status – and desire to show off their power – is translated into pleasure, often through sex-based consumption. Examining how such actions can help nurture and reinstate the bonds of 'homosociality' that are of central importance in Mexican daily life, the authors explore the implications of these sexualized homecomings for the regional epidemiology of HIV and for approaches to its prevention.

## Mobility and work

The pursuit of work is a key driver of mobility both across international borders and within countries, a situation that is examined in greater depth in the chapters in the final section of the book. In many cases, the structure of the labour migration process results in long term separations between regular partners, detachment from stabilizing norms, and increased peer and other pressures to engage in particular forms of sexuality. This is well demonstrated in Mark Hunter's chapter (Chapter 11), which builds on the emerging literature on the political economy of intimacy in the context of HIV and AIDS in South Africa. Hunter examines the ways in which recent and interconnected trends of rising unemployment, social inequalities, reduced marriage rates, and widespread labour migration of women as well as men can impact upon ideas concerning – and the practice of – intimacy and sexual relationships.

The concern with long-term migration and HIV risk is clearly evident in Kennedy Ondimu's analysis (Chapter 12) of the impact of the poor living and working conditions faced by migrant labourers on a Kenyan tea plantation. Ondimu emphasizes the norms and expectations that encourage men to pursue multiple relationships, and the particular constraints faced by single and divorced women. Many of the latter are unable to rely on traditional support networks, and use unprotected transactional sex as a way of securing economic gain and protection from physical violence. In the next chapter (Chapter 13), Lorraine van Blerk provides a detailed discussion of the ways in which economic circumstances can influence decisions to move amongst young women sex workers in Ethiopia. She examines the mobility pathways that lead young women into sex work, the often abusive and high-risk nature of sexual interactions under these circumstances, and the pressures young women face to move to secure work once it is suspected they are HIV positive.

Despite such evidence linking HIV transmission and labour-related mobility, however, it is vital to recognize the heterogeneity of mobile populations, and the conditions under which they move and in which they work. Holly Wardlow's account of HIV risk in Papua New Guinea (Chapter 14) provides an important overview of the ways in which population mobility has changed over time, giving rise to different patterns of sexual networking, which in turn have a very different impact on HIV vulnerability within different communities and in different sectors. Wardlow shows how the different meanings invested in the act of migration can influence HIV risk and vulnerability. She demonstrates that in some areas labour migration has become an integral part of a masculine identity that encourages men to demonstrate their independence from community norms and expectations through extramarital liaisons, how in other areas, well-intentioned labour migration policies have given rise to unanticipated consequences that increase HIV vulnerability a generation later, and how local labour migration policies in the mining industry contribute to patterns of sexual networking and HIV-related risk in ways that are far different from those observed elsewhere, and may in fact act as protective factors against HIV transmission.

In many countries where HIV is primarily transmitted through heterosexual sex, it is increasingly recognized that marriage can pose substantial risk, particularly for women whose husbands work away from home. Daniel Jordan Smith (Chapter 15) looks at this question from the points of view of both husbands and wives, providing important insights into the changing nature of marriage in Igbo-speaking areas of Nigeria. He argues that men's extramarital liaisons must be understood within the context of the wider structural opportunities and social circumstances in a predominantly sex-segregated social context that encourages and rewards such behaviour. While this clearly applies to men involved in migrant labour, Jordan Smith makes the important point that it can also apply to men who live with their wives, since social and cultural norms afford married men considerably more day-to-day mobility and associated freedoms than those available to married women. This important chapter raises key issues concerning the transformation of the ways in which men's and women's (often differing) ideas and expectations concerning romance, intimacy and marriage can actually undermine women's power within sexual relationships, making it difficult for women to negotiate condom use even when their husbands' infidelities are known.

Finally, Xiushi Yang (Chapter 16) examines the rapid increase in HIV prevalence in China, and explores the ways in which different forms of labour migration can pose different levels of HIV risk and vulnerability. Particular focus here is placed upon the contrasting experiences of temporary migrants, permanent migrants, and non-migrants and the various levels of social and economic rights available to each under China's household registration system. Using sophisticated quantitative research methods, the study described in Yang's chapter once again demonstrates the importance of social integration and rights for decreasing HIV risk and vulnerability.

Taken together, the various chapters of *Mobility, Sexuality and AIDS* provide a broad overview of the issues emerging from recent research on the health and wellbeing of mobile populations in general, and the relationship between sexuality, HIV, AIDS and population mobility in particular. As the chapters clearly demonstrate, understanding the heterogeneous nature of mobile populations and of experiences of mobility can help focus attention on the ways in which others perceive and respond to different populations. The editors hope the book will help move thinking about population mobility and its relation to HIV away from the fear that outsiders might bring infectious diseases – and also beyond country contexts. We hope it will increase understanding of how – whether it is chosen or enforced, whether for work or for pleasure – mobility may affect sexuality and sense of self. In particular, we hope that readers will come away with more understanding of how social and cultural constructions of sexuality help shape HIV risk and vulnerability.

## References

Apostolopoulos, Y., and Sonmez, S. (2007) *Population Mobility and Infectious Diseases*. New York: Springer.

Campbell, C. (1997) 'Migrancy, Masculine Identities and AIDS: the Psychosocial Context of HIV Transmission on the South Africa Gold Mines', *Social Science & Medicine*, 45(2): 273–81.

Coker, R. (2003) 'Migration, Public Health and Compulsory Screening for TB and HIV', *Asylum and Migration Working Paper 1*. London: IPPR.

Farmer, P. (1999) AIDS and Social Scientists: Critical Reflections . In Becker, C., Dozon, J., Obbo, C., and Toure, M. (eds) *Experiencing and Understanding AIDS in Africa*. Paris: èditions Karthala.

Herdt, G. (1997) Sexual Cultures and Population Movement: Implications for AIDS/ STDs . In *Sexual Cultures and Migration in the Era of AIDS: Anthropological and Demographic Perspectives*. Oxford: Clarendon Press.

Ingram, A. (2005) 'The New Geopolitics of Disease: Between Global Health and Global Security', *Geopolitics*, 10(3): 522–45.

Jatrana, S., Graham, E., and Boyle, P. (2005) 'Introduction: Understanding Migration and Health in Asia'. In Jatrana, S., Toyota, M., and Yeoh, S. A. (eds) *Migration and Health in Asia*. London: Routledge.

Kimmel, M. S., and Plante, R. F. (2004) *Sexualities: Identities, Behaviors, and Society*. New York: Lancaster Press.

Kraut, A. M. (1995) *Silent Travellers: Genes, Germs and the 'Immigrant Menace'*. Baltimore, Massachusetts: John Hopkins University Press.

Lurie, M., Williams, B. G., Khangelani, Z., Mkaya-Mwamburi, D., Garnett, G. P. Sturm, A. W., Sweat, M. D., Gittelsohn, J., and Abdool Karim, S. S. (2003) 'The Impact of Migration on HIV-1 Transmission in South Africa: A Study of Nonmigrant Men and Their Partners', *Sexually Transmitted Diseases*, 30(2): 149–56.

Manalansan, M. F. (2006) Queer Intersections: Sexuality and Gender in Migration Studies . *International Migration Review*, 40(1): 224–249.

Parker, R. (2001) Sexuality, Culture and Power in HIV/AIDS Research . *Annual Review of Anthropology*, 30: 163–179.

Parker, R., and Aggleton, P. (2007) *Culture, Society and Sexuality: A Reader*. London: Routledge.

Parker, R., Barbosa, R. M., and Aggleton, P. (2000) *Framing the Sexual Subject: The Politics of Gender, Sexuality and Power*. Berkeley, California: University of California Press.

Patton, C. (2002) *Globalizing AIDS*. Minneapolis, Minnesota: University of Minnesota Press

Prins, G. (2004) 'AIDS and Global Security', *International Affairs*, 80(5): 931–52.

# Migration and HIV infection

## What do data from destination countries show?

*Islene Araujo de Carvalho, Mary Haour-Knipe and Karl L. Dehne*

The relationship between migration and epidemic infectious diseases has long been a subject of concern, as well as the object of efforts to stop the spread of diseases. In recent years, and as the issue of international migration has moved to the forefront of national and international agendas, the link between HIV infection and migration, in particular, has raised the interest of researchers and policy-makers. It has been hypothesized that migrants are at increased risk of exposure to HIV, and to transmission of infection, due to an increase in HIV-related vulnerability due to migration, such as the weakening of protective social norms during the migration process, and lack of information about – and protection from – HIV at destination (c.f. Decosas *et al.* 1995; International Organization for Migration 2005). Compelling evidence remains scarce, however. This chapter attempts to address this lack by examining the epidemiological evidence available about HIV infection among one group, international migrants in countries of destination

## Methods

A review of available evidence was conducted using PubMed, with the following search terms: 'HIV Infection' and 'Emigration' and 'Immigration'. Included were all studies that focused on migrants in destination countries; that reported HIV prevalence, related information on patterns of HIV transmission, and/or place where the infection was acquired (i.e. in country of origin or in destination country); and that were published between 1998 and 2008. A few additional studies were identified through contacts with offices of the International Organization for Migration and with researchers known to be working on the subject. Studies conducted specifically among internal migrants and internally displaced persons, as well as among people affected by humanitarian emergencies, such as refugees, were excluded (see Spiegel *et al.* 2007 for a recent review concerning such populations, as well as Roberts and Patel, this volume).

## Findings

Seventy-seven articles were retrieved, of which 27 were retained according to the inclusion criteria. The majority of studies had been carried out in Europe or North America, with a few conducted in Asia. Among the 27 studies included here, 12 contained pertinent information on HIV infection rates among migrants in destination countries. Most made comparisons with non-migrant populations in the country in which the study had been carried out, reported on transmission patterns, and included data on whether transmission may have occurred before or after migration. The majority of the studies with data on HIV prevalence among migrants had a cross-sectional design, surveying individuals at one point in time in order to gather information on health status, including HIV status. Only two relevant cohort studies were identified, and no such study comparing a group exposed to migration with a group not thus exposed in order to determine if there might be any differences in HIV incidence between the two. The studies were descriptive rather than analytical – none attempted to test hypothesises regarding the role of migration as a potential determinant of HIV infection. The prevalence studies retained are presented in Table 1.1.

### *Rates of HIV infection among migrants*

Data from 12 studies conducted among migrants in North America, Europe, Asia and the Middle East are summarized in Table 1.1. Although the numbers are to be treated with caution for reasons discussed later in this chapter, several of the studies indicate higher rates of HIV infection for migrants than for the general population in the destination country. In the USA, for example, and among all HIV cases residing in one county in the state of Washington, HIV was 2.8 times more frequent among foreign-born Blacks than among native-born Blacks (1.7 per cent and 0.6 per cent, respectively) (Kent 2005).

A different US study, carried out in Los Angeles among foreign-born clients of clinics for sexually transmitted infections (STIs), reported that overall, the former were *not* more likely to be HIV positive than were US-born clients, although HIV prevalence was higher among clients from North Africa and the Middle East (3.3 per cent) and among those from the Caribbean and West Indies (2.9 per cent, compared with 0.4 per cent for all foreign-born clients) (Harawa *et al.* 2002). In Canada, one of the classic studies in the field of migration and HIV found prevalence to be higher among Haitian migrants in Canada than among Canadian natives. Those who had arrived more recently, or who had travelled to Haiti in the previous five years had particularly high infection rates (Adrien *et al.* 1999).

In Europe, a cross-sectional community-based survey carried out among self-defined Black Africans in three communities in England found HIV prevalence to be higher than among the general UK population: overall HIV prevalence in

Table 1.1 Studies of HIV prevalence among migrants in destination countries

| Destination country | Author | Year data gathered | N | Population | HIV prevalence (%) Migrants (in year data gathered) | Destination country (2007)* | Country of origin (2007)*,** |
|---|---|---|---|---|---|---|---|
| USA | Kent | 1995–2003 | 3,383 | All HIV+ cases residing in King County, WA, at time of study; HIV prevalence calculated for foreign-born blacks | Foreign-born blacks: 1.7 Native-born blacks: 0.6 All county residents: 0.3 | 0.6 | Ethiopia: 2.1 Kenya: 7.1–8.5 |
| USA | Harawa | 1993–1995 | 61,120 | STD clients in 7 Los Angeles Public Heath Centers (country of birth) | Born in: - Central America/Mexico: 1.6 - Sub-Saharan Africa: 2.2 - North Africa/Middle East: 3.3 - Caribbean/West Indies: 2.9 - East Asia/Pacific Islands: 0.5 Overall clinic attendees: 0.4 | 0.6 | Latin America: 0.5 Mexico: 0.3 Sub-Saharan Africa: 5.0 North Africa/Middle East: 0.3 Caribbean: 1.1 East Asia: 0.1 |
| Canada | Adrien et al. | 1994–1996 | 5,039 | People born in Haiti or with one parent born in Haiti, recruited in 7 clinics | Montreal residents of Haitian origin: 1.3 | 0.4 | Haiti: 2.2 |
| UK | Sadler et al. | 2004 | Total: 1608 Agreed to HIV test: 1006 | Black Africans recruited in 3 communities (self-identified as being of 'black African ethnicity') | Overall Black Africans: 14 (M: 13.1; F: 15.0) East AfricaM: 21.8; F: 25.4 Horn of AfricaM: 2.7; F: 4.2 Southern AfricaM: 18.2; F: 33.3 Central AfricaM: 7.1; F: 11.4 Western AfricaM: 7.0; F: 6.2 | 0.2 | Sub-Saharan Africa: 5.0 Uganda: 5.4 Zimbabwe: 15.3 |

Table 1.1 (continued)

| Destination country | Author | Year data gathered | N | Population | HIV prevalence (%) Migrants (in year data gathered) | Destination country (2007)* | Country of origin (2007)*,** |
|---|---|---|---|---|---|---|---|
| Netherlands | Gras et al. | 1997–1998 | 1660 | Immigrants in Amsterdam self-identified as Surinamese, Antillean and sub-Saharan African | Surinamese, Antilleans, sub-Saharan Africans: 1.1 | 0.2 | Suriname: 2.4 Sub-Saharan Africa: 5.0 |
| Netherlands | Stolte et al. | 1997–1998 | 1474 | Self-identified Afro-Surinamese, Dutch-Antillean. Ghanaians & Nigerians from previous study (Gras et al. 1999) | West Africans: 1.4 Dutch-Antillean: 1.8 Afro-Surinamese: 0.5 | 0.2 | Ghana: 1.9 Nigeria: 3.1 Suriname: 2.4 |
| Spain | Vall Mayans et al. | 2000 | 1453 | Clients of Barcelona STD clinic | Immigrants: 1.8 Residents: 1.7 | 0.5 | … |
| Spain | Castilla et al. | 2000 | 8861 | National and non-Spanish subjects voluntarily tested at 18 STI/HIV clinics in 16 cities in Spain | Country of origin in: Western Europe: 2.7 Central & Eastern Europe: 1.7 Latin America: 1.7 Sub-Saharan Africa: 8.4 North Africa: 2.4 Others: 1.2 Spanish clients: 1.8 | 0.5 | Western & Central Europe: 0.3 Latin America: 0.5 Sub-Saharan Africa: 5.0 North Africa/Middle East: 0.3 |
| Italy | Spizzichino et al. | 1993–1999 | 353 | All foreign male-to-female transsexual sex workers who presented for HIV testing at one hospital in Rome | Foreign transsexual sex workers: 38.2 | 0.4 | Colombia: 0.6 Brazil: 0.6 |
| Thailand | Wiwanitkit and Waenlor | Not stated (prior to 2002) | 250 | Myanmar migrants in Southern Thailand | Recently arrived migrants: 3.2 | 1.4 | Myanmar: 0.7 |

(Continued on next page)

Table 1.1 (continued)

| Destination country | Author | Year data gathered | N | Population | HIV prevalence (%) | | |
|---|---|---|---|---|---|---|---|
| | | | | | Migrants (in year data gathered) | Destination country (2007)* | Country of origin (2007)*,** |
| Thailand | Srithanavi-boonchai | 1999 | 429 | Myanmar labour migrants in Chiang Mai province, Thailand | Ethnic Shan migrant workers: 4.9 | 1.4 | Myanmar: 0.7 |
| Kuwait | Akhtar & Mohammad | 1997–2006 | 2,328,582 | Migrant workers entering Kuwait (data from routine medical exams, which include HIV testing) | Entering migrant workers: 0.021 | Available estimates: under 0.2 | India: 0.3 Bangladesh: <0.1 Sri-Lanka: <0.1 Egypt: <0.1 Indonesia: 0.2 |

*Source: 2008 Report on the Global AIDS epidemic, UNAIDS/WHO, July 2008. Data are given as a rough point of reference, but should not be used to draw firm conclusions since the groups studied are not necessarily comparable in age, sex or profession, among other variables and not representative of the general population in either country of origin or destination

**Specific countries are listed where given in source article

the migrant population studied was 14 per cent, with significant differences by region of origin and by sex. Prevalence was higher among UK residents from East and Southern Africa, and – with the exception of Western Africa – among female migrants (Sadler *et al.* 2007). Studies carried out in the Netherlands and using methods similar to those of the UK study (voluntary HIV testing carried out as part of a larger study of members of ethnic minority communities approached in public places such as shopping areas and community events) also found HIV prevalence to be somewhat higher among migrants in comparison with the general Dutch population (Gras *et al.* 1999), especially among migrants from West Africa and the Dutch Antilles (Stolte *et al.* 2003).

In Barcelona, Spain, in a study among presumably higher-risk STI patients, on the other hand, HIV prevalence was reportedly similar for immigrants and native residents (1.8 per cent for immigrants vs 1.7 per cent for Spanish) (Vall-Mayans *et al.* 2002). Also in Spain, examination of data from clinics offering voluntary, free, confidential and often anonymous counselling and testing for STI/HIV in 16 large cities found that nearly one-third of those who presented for testing were 'of foreign origin'. At 8.4 per cent, HIV prevalence among migrant clients from sub-Sahara Africa was higher than among those who came from other regions or among Spanish subjects (1.8 per cent among the latter, for example) (Castilla *et al.* 2002). A study from Italy also focused on a specific sub-group of migrants potentially at high risk: HIV prevalence was found to be relatively high among foreign, mainly Colombian and Brazilian, transsexual sex workers presenting for HIV testing at a specialized hospital in Rome (Spizzichino *et al.* 2001).

Only two studies of Asian migrants were found. Both came from Thailand, a country that receives large numbers of migrant workers from neighbouring countries. HIV prevalence was found to be relatively high among migrants from Myanmar in that country, both in the Southern Region, an area with a high density of Burmese fishermen (Wiwanitkit and Waenlor 2002) and among ethnic Shan Burmese migrant workers further north in Chang Mai province. Figures for the latter were almost double that of comparison groups of Thais (pregnant women and military recruits) in the same province (Srithanaviboonchai *et al.* 2002).

Finally, one relevant study was found from the Middle East, where data gathered over 10 years of mandatory HIV testing of migrant workers entering Kuwait, most of whom were from South Asian countries, showed an HIV infection rate of 0.021 per cent, substantially lower than the national estimates for Kuwait (Akhtar and Mohammad 2008).

The last column of Table 1.1 lists HIV prevalence in the countries from which the migrants in each of the studies came. Although here, too, extreme caution is warranted in interpreting the data, an intriguing pattern emerges: in most cases HIV prevalence among migrants from high prevalence countries is lower than the national prevalence in their countries or regions of origin. Among migrants from relatively low prevalence countries the situation is the opposite: HIV pre-valence among the migrants is higher than the overall national prevalence in their country of origin (examples are Mexicans in the USA, migrants from North Africa and Middle East in the USA and Spain, and migrant workers from Myanmar in Thailand). There are some exceptions to this pattern: in particular, migrants from sub-Saharan Africa reached through random community sampling in the UK, and also through clinics in Spain for voluntary counselling and testing of HIV (and in some instances also for other STIs), were found to have higher rates of HIV in destination countries than in countries of origin.

### Characteristics of HIV transmission

Modes of HIV transmission among migrant populations tend to reflect modes of transmission in their countries of origin, and may thus be different from those observed among other populations in their countries of destination. For example, one of the American studies listed in Table 1.1 found that heterosexual transmission accounted for the majority of cases among foreign-born Blacks, but for only 12 per cent of native-born Blacks in the community studied (Kent 2005).

Several studies from European countries (not all of which appear in Table 1.1 since they do not contain prevalence data) have examined the question of modes of transmission among migrant populations. Although the groups most affected by HIV in native Europeans are men who have sex with men and injecting drug users, heterosexual transmission has consistently been found to be more frequent among migrants. For example, an analysis of data concerning African communities in the UK showed that 88 per cent of the HIV infections among Black Africans in that country was acquired heterosexually. The next most common route of infection was mother to child transmission (Sinka et al. 2003).

A cross-sectional case-control study carried out in Italy, similarly, found that immigrants with HIV from outside the European Union (EU) were more likely to have been infected heterosexually or prenatally than were Italian and EU patients of the same age and sex (Manfredi et al. 2001). And in Greece, 41 per cent of the 750 migrants reported to the Hellenic Centre for Infectious Diseases Control between 1989 and 2003 were classified as having been infected through heterosexual contact – and 19 per cent through male homosexual contact – whereas the proportions were practically inversed for the almost 5000 Greek HIV-positive cases (16 per cent infected through heterosexual contact and 50 per cent men who have sex with men). The same study reported that the percentage of injecting drug users among people originating from other countries was almost twofold that among Greeks (7.7 per cent vs 3.2 per cent) (Nikolopoulos et al. 2005).

The studies described in the previous paragraph analyzed modes of transmission among migrants already known to be HIV infected. At least two of the studies presented in Table 1.1 carried out HIV testing among migrant general populations (in other words among the ordinary 'person in the street' in communities where many migrants live) and then examined modes of infection among those who were found to be HIV positive. In the Netherlands, a large-scale study that offered HIV testing in immigrant communities found 18 HIV infections among the 1660 people tested, for which same-sex sexual contact (for men) and sex with an injecting drug user were reported to be the main modes of transmission (Gras *et al.* 1999). The Spanish study that looked at data from clinics offering free Voluntary Counselling and Testing (VCT) also revealed some surprising findings concerning mode of HIV transmission among the 59 non-Spanish patients found to be HIV positive: as in other studies, heterosexual transmission predominated among migrants from Africa; but injecting drug use and homosexual transmission predominated for patients from Latin America; relatively low HIV prevalence was found among Latin American women who work in the sex industry, but high prevalence was found among heterosexual women from northern Africa not known to be involved in sex work (Castilla *et al.* 2002).

These studies begin to reveal some of the complex patterns underlying the raw epidemiological data, as do the studies that are beginning to focus more finely on sub-groups of migrants, such as on migrant men who have sex with men for example (c.f. Dougan *et al.* 2005).

### Where infection occurs

The literature reviewed gives uneven evidence concerning whether infections among migrants may have taken place in the country of origin, in transit, or the destination country. A first basic factor is clearly how long the migrant has been in the destination country. Thus among Myanmar migrants who had been in Thailand for less than a month, the infections had also almost certainly occurred before their arrival in Thailand or possibly in transit (Wiwanitkit and Waenlor 2002).

Some of the studies of HIV prevalence among migrants presented in Table 1.1 address the question of where infection might have taken place. The study of HIV-positive immigrants from Central America and Mexico living in Los Angeles, for example, concluded that most had undoubtedly acquired their HIV infection after they arrived since most had migrated many years previously and at a relatively young age (Harawa *et al.* 2002). Similarly, although the numbers are very small, the study among migrants in Amsterdam presents evidence that suggests they acquired the infection after they migrated to Europe: among the 18 people who tested positive, nine had reported a previous negative test, six of which were carried out after they had arrived (Gras *et al.* 1999). The authors of the study of HIV infection among people of foreign origin voluntarily tested in Spain also noted that it was highly probable that those who had had a previous negative test in the same clinic – at least 15 per cent of the sample – became infected after their arrival, and cite another study carried out in Barcelona that estimated that more than one-quarter of the immigrants with AIDS became infected after their arrival (García de Olaya *et al.* 2000 cited in Castilla *et al.* 2002).

Along similar lines, but on a different continent and under quite different circumstances, migration has been identified as a risk factor for HIV in Pakistan.

In a major migrant-sending area in the south of the country, 73 per cent of the HIV/AIDS cases reported to the Sindh AIDS Control Programme between 1996 and 1998 were among former overseas workers who had been deported from Gulf countries because of their HIV status.[1] A further 7 per cent were wives of deported workers. Since HIV testing is required by the destination countries before arrival, and would-be workers will only be granted a residence permit if they test negative, the evidence thus suggests that infections occurred after migration (Shah *et al.* 1999).

Data on the relative importance of either pre- or post-migration HIV infection is available from studies in Israel, a country which also requires HIV testing of entering immigrants. Epidemic modelling in that country suggested that adult HIV incidence among Ethiopian immigrants was between three and 11 infections per 1000 uninfected persons and year, while incidence in this group before immigration in Ethiopia was estimated at between 12 and 22 infections (Kaplan *et al.* 1998).

In the Swiss cohort study (a long-running study that includes approximately 70 per cent of those living with AIDS in Switzerland) clinical data concerning migrants attending one of the larger participating clinics were examined. CD4 cell count decline over time, and plasma HIV RNA levels, led the authors to conclude that 70 per cent of the patients from sub-Saharan Africa and 50 per cent of those from Southeast Asia had most probably been infected before entry (Staehelin *et al.* 2004). Similarly, in the UK, analysis of the data available on country of likely infection, as well as of ethnicity, showed that up to the end of 2001, 21 per cent of all HIV infections in that country were probably acquired in Africa, including about 67 per cent of those acquired through heterosexual sex. Records showed that 61 per cent of the latter were Black African. The authors add, however, that the information on the subject is far from being complete: there was no ethnicity data available for over one-quarter of those listed as having been infected in Africa (Sinka *et al.* 2003).

Finally, a number of studies have found evidence that visits to countries of origin could put migrants at significant risk for contracting HIV. Of the studies presented in Table 1.1, HIV prevalence doubled among Haitians in Canada who frequently travelled to Haiti (Adrien *et al.* 1999). Similarly, among Surinamese, Antilleans and Africans in the Netherlands, the risk of being HIV infected was associated with travelling to and having sex in the country of origin (Gras *et al.* 1999).

A few studies have specifically examined sexual risk-taking behaviour during travel to countries of origin. In Asia, for example, Vietnamese migrants living in Australia have been found to put themselves at risk during visits home (O'Connor *et al.* 2007). In Europe, Fenton and colleagues found that amongst 756 Africans residing in the UK, almost half (43 per cent of the men and 46 per cent of the women) had visited their home country in the previous five years, in proportions that varied by country of origin, length of residence in the UK and level of education and employment. Forty per cent of the men and 21 per cent of women acquired a new sexual partner while travelling abroad (Fenton *et al.*

2001). And in a similar study among 798 Surinamese and 227 Antillean migrants in Amsterdam, 38 per cent of the men and 42 per cent of the women had visited their homeland in the previous five years. As in the UK, visits were more frequent among migrants who had been abroad longer, who were employed, and who had higher levels of education. Of migrants visiting their homeland, 47 per cent of the men and 11 per cent of the women acquired a local sexual partner while abroad, and of these one-third of the men and half of the women had unprotected sex (Kramer *et al.* 2005).

## Discussion

A first finding from the review concerns the paucity of well-designed epidemiological studies involving international migrants. Most of the studies identified using the criteria described at the beginning of this chapter came from Europe and North America. While time and resource constraints did not permit searching other electronic databases, reviewing many articles other than in English, or contacting a broader range of researchers on HIV and migration, we believe this paucity of studies reflects existing research. It also reflects testing policies concerning migrants. The lack of data from Asia and the Middle East, for example, can be explained by the fact that most HIV testing of migrants in these regions is carried out as part of migrant worker health screenings either before departure or upon arrival. Most is undertaken by the private sector, often at the request of employers or destination country governments,[2] and the results are not published.

As for Africa, no study among international labour migrants appeared in the search. A good deal of excellent research concerning population mobility and HIV has been carried out on that continent, but most of the studies concentrate on internal migrants or mixed flows of migrants, refugees and short-term travellers. A few studies have been carried out among European and North American expatriates in African countries, but after their return to Europe and the USA.

A second finding concerns the overall quality of the studies that were found. Only a few fulfilled minimum criteria for statistically sound comparisons between migrant and native populations: confidence intervals around point estimates were rarely provided, and some reports failed to provide information on basic characteristics such as migrants' age, sex and country of origin. Several studies were based on small samples from selected geographical areas that were unlikely to be representative of either migrant or non-migrant populations. Some included no comparison group, or uncritically attempted to compare small surveys with national data. Another major issue concerns variability in the way the 'migrant' group was defined. Different studies use time since migration, nationality, country of birth, or self-described ethnic affiliation as the defining criterion making comparison between countries hazardous at best.

These methodological considerations aside, several important findings emerge. Some of the studies reviewed showed higher HIV prevalence among migrants than among non-migrants in destination countries on several different continents (c.f. Adrien *et al.* 1999; Kent 2005; Sadler *et al.* 2007; Srithanaviboonchai *et al.* 2002). Such findings are hardly surprising given that many of the migrants came from countries with generalized epidemics, and may well have acquired HIV before they left. Other studies, on the contrary, showed infection rates that were not higher among migrants as compared with the native population (c.f. Castilla *et al.* 2002), or possibly even lower (c.f. Akhtar and Mohammad 2008), which might suggest similar or lower levels of risk. Whatever the findings, such studies are subject to many biases, including economic and health-related self-selection before migration, the effect of HIV-related travel restrictions which may prevent would-be migrants who know they are HIV infected to present for testing, and selection in the destination country. As one of the reports reviewed pointed out, studies of migrant clients of clinics that offer free and easy access to VCT and to treatment of other STIs may over-represent those with difficulties in access to other health facilities (Castilla *et al.* 2002). In addition, most-at-risk populations, such as sex workers, injecting drug users, or people with STIs, are over-represented among the migrant populations analyzed in several studies, especially when they are carried out in health care settings (Castilla *et al.* 2002; Harawa *et al.* 2002; c.f. Spizzichino *et al.* 2001; Vall-Mayans *et al.* 2002). All of these factors make generalizations about the strength of the association between migration and HIV status hazardous. Overall the evidence does not suggest that being a migrant or a foreigner in a developed country is per se associated with higher levels of HIV infection. The situation is more complex than that.

The modes of transmission reported and their association with likely country of infection provide some insight into the possible links between migration and HIV, and into the risk behaviours, situations, and environments migrants may encounter in countries of origin and destination. Thus, people from countries of origin with high prevalence may bring the heterosexual transmission that predominates in their countries with them, be it by methodological bias (being registered as a case of 'heterosexual transmission' simply on the basis of coming from a high-prevalence country), or by actually contracting and transmitting HIV heterosexually when they follow migration patterns created by historical links between their countries of origin and of destination. When appropriate prevention and care is lacking they may also experience perinatal transmission in destination countries.

The data concerning HIV transmission through same-sex sexual relations among migrants, in particular, illustrate many of the complexities of the migration process and of gathering and interpreting data about migrant populations. Gay and other homosexually active men who are able to migrate may do so in order to live a sexual life style that is difficult to pursue in their home community (see Carrillo, this volume), miss out on HIV prevention as they do so, and thus become disproportionately affected. Or, to suggest a plausible bias in the opposite direction, stigmatization and stereotypes may cause health workers to underestimate and under-diagnose HIV infection among migrant gay and other homosexual men on the false assumption that there are no such men among a given migrant group.

Some of the studies discussed in this chapter report higher HIV prevalence among female migrants, and some define subgroups of migrant women as particularly severely affected. We were unable to systematically elaborate on such differences here. They merit much further exploration.

Another important finding of the review is that migrants do risk infection after arrival in destination countries. The review clearly showed that long-term Central American migrants in the USA, migrants from various countries in Amsterdam and Barcelona, Ethiopians in Israel and various subgroups of ethnic minority communities in the UK had all acquired HIV in the destination country. Some of the more surprising findings from among Surinamese in the Netherlands, Latina women and men and Northern African women in Spain, and some of the migrants in Greece also suggest the acquisition of new risk behaviours in countries of destination. The implications of such findings obviously include the often-cited need to provide migrants with culturally sensitive and locally relevant prevention information, as well as access to appropriate counselling, care and support, as soon as possible after their arrival.

## Conclusion

This chapter has shown both the complexity of the epidemiology of HIV in the context of migration, and the paucity of high-quality data. It has demonstrated many linkages, revealed gaps and problems, and begun to highlight what might be effective in addressing these. Quantitative data on HIV infection among migrants in destination countries, and on modes of transmission and likely country of infection, only provide a glimpse of the sexual and drug-related behaviours, vulnerability context and service needs that underlie these figures, however. Further research, including qualitative and historical studies, will need to be conducted to better understand migrants' motivations and experiences.

The potential for further spread of HIV linked to population mobility – including from and to migrants – is real, especially where significant numbers of people migrate when already infected and/or when new high-risk behaviours and situations are acquired and encountered at destination. Bridges exist, both between migrants and host country populations, and between migrants and people in countries of origin, for example, during visits home. Policies and programmes will need to be developed to address these risks and vulnerabilities. Such programmes would be better grounded, however, if the evidence on which they were based was improved.

## Acknowledgements

The authors would like to thank Rosilyne Borland for providing useful comments on this text, and Lucas Hallimani and Mudassar Abad for sharing additional references.

## Notes

1 Foreign nationals in the Gulf States are required to renew their work permit and their HIV test every 2 years. Anyone found HIV positive is immediately deported to the country of origin.
2 For a discussion of the question of mandatory HIV testing of migrant labourers, see 'Report of the International Task Team on HIV-related Travel Restrictions: Findings and Recommendations', available at www.data.unaids.org/pub/Report/2008/20081017_itt_report_travel_restrictions_en.pdf (accessed 3 March 2009).

## References

Adrien, A., Leaune, V., Remis, R. S., Boivin, J. F., Rud, E., Duperval, R., and Noel, G. E. (1999) 'Migration and HIV: an epidemiological study of Montrealers of Haitian origin', *International Journal of STD & AIDS*, *10*(4), 237–42.

Akhtar, S., and Mohammad, H. G. (2008) 'Spectral analysis of HIV seropositivity among migrant workers entering Kuwait', *BMC Infectious Diseases*, *8*, 37.

Castilla, J., Sobrino, P., and del Amo, J. (2002) 'HIV infection among people of foreign origin voluntarily tested in Spain: a comparison with national subjects', *Sexually Transmitted Infections*, *78*(4), 250–54.

Decosas, J., Kane, F., Anarfi, J. K., Sodji, K. D., and Wagner, H. U. (1995) 'Migration and AIDS', *Lancet*, *346*(8978), 826–28.

Dougan, S., Elford, J., Rice, B., Brown, A. E., Sinka, K., Evans, B. G., Gill, O. N., and Fenton, K. A. (2005) 'Epidemiology of HIV among black and minority ethnic men who have sex with men in England and Wales', *Sexually Transmitted Infections*, *81*(4), 345–50.

Fenton, K. A., Chinouya, M., Davidson, O., and Copas, A. (2001) 'HIV transmission risk among sub-Saharan Africans in London travelling to their countries of origin', *AIDS*, *15*(11), 1442–45.

Gras, M. J., Weide, J. F., Langendam, M. W., Coutinho, R. A., and van den, H. A. (1999) 'HIV prevalence, sexual risk behaviour and sexual mixing patterns among migrants in Amsterdam, The Netherlands', *AIDS*, *13*(14), 1953–62.

Harawa, N. T., Bingham, T. A., Cochran, S. D., Greenland, S., and Cunningham, W. E. (2002) 'HIV prevalence among foreign- and US-born clients of public STD clinics', *American Journal of Public Health*, *92*(12), 1958–63.

International Organization for Migration (2005) *World Migration 2005: Costs and Benefits of International Migration*. Geneva: IOM.

Kaplan, E. H., Kedem, E., and Pollack, S. (1998) 'HIV incidence in Ethiopian immigrants to Israel', *Journal of Acquired Immune Deficiency Syndrome and Human Retrovirology*, *17*(5), 465–69.

Kent, J. B. (2005) 'Impact of foreign-born persons on HIV diagnosis rates among Blacks in King County, Washington', *AIDS Education and Prevention*, *17*(6 Suppl B), 60–67.

Kramer, M. A., van den, H. A., Coutinho, R. A., and Prins, M. (2005) 'Sexual risk behaviour among Surinamese and Antillean migrants travelling to their countries of origin', *Sexually Transmitted Infections*, *81*(6), 508–10.

Manfredi, R., Calza, L., and Chiodo, F. (2001) 'HIV disease among immigrants coming to Italy from outside of the European Union: a case-control study of epidemiological and clinical features', *Epidemiology and Infection*, *127*(3), 527–33.

Nikolopoulos, G., Arvanitis, M., Masgala, A., and Paraskeva, D. (2005) 'Migration and HIV epidemic in Greece', *European Journal of Public Health*, *15*(3), 296–99.

O'Connor, C. C., Wen, L. M., Rissel, C., and Shaw, M. (2007) 'Sexual behaviour and risk in Vietnamese men living in metropolitan Sydney', *Sexually Transmitted Infections, 83* (2), 147–50.

Sadler, K. E., McGarrigle, C. A., Elam, G., Ssanyu-Sseruma, W., Davidson, O., Nichols, T., Mercey, D., Parry, J. V., and Fenton, K. A. (2007) 'Sexual behaviour and HIV infection in black-Africans in England: results from the Mayisha II survey of sexual attitudes and lifestyles', *Sexually Transmitted Infections, 83*(7), 523–29.

Shah, S. A., Khan, O. A., Kristensen, S., and Vermund, S. H. (1999) 'HIV-infected workers deported from the Gulf States: impact on Southern Pakistan', *International Journal of STD & AIDS, 10*(12), 812–14.

Sinka, K., Mortimer, J., Evans, B., and Morgan, D. (2003) 'Impact of the HIV epidemic in sub-Saharan Africa on the pattern of HIV in the UK', *AIDS, 17*(11), 1683–90.

Spiegel, P. B., Bennedsen, A. R., Claass, J., Bruns, L., Patterson, N., Yiweza, D., and Schilperoord, M. (2007) 'Prevalence of HIV infection in conflict-affected and displaced people in seven sub-Saharan African countries: a systematic review', *Lancet, 369*(9580), 2187–95.

Spizzichino, L., Zaccarelli, M., Rezza, G., Ippolito, G., Antinori, A., and Gattari, P. (2001) 'HIV infection among foreign transsexual sex workers in Rome: prevalence, behavior patterns, and seroconversion rates', *Sexually Transmitted Diseases, 28*(7), 405–11.

Srithanaviboonchai, K., Choi, K. H., van, G. F., Hudes, E. S., Visaruratana, S., and Mandel, J. S. (2002) 'HIV-1 in ethnic Shan migrant workers in northern Thailand', *AIDS, 16*(6), 929–31.

Staehelin, C., Egloff, N., Rickenbach, M., Kopp, C., and Furrer, H. (2004) 'Migrants from sub-Saharan Africa in the Swiss HIV Cohort Study: a single center study of epidemiologic migration-specific and clinical features', *AIDS Patient Care & STDS, 18*(11), 665–75.

Stolte, I. G., Gras, M., Van Benthem, B. H., Coutinho, R. A., and van den Hoek, J. A. (2003) 'HIV testing behaviour among heterosexual migrants in Amsterdam', *AIDS Care, 15*(4), 563–74.

Vall-Mayans, M., Arellano, E., Armengol, P., Escriba, J. M., Loureiro, E., Saladie, P., Sanz, B., Saravanya, M., Vall, M., and Villena, M. J. (2002) '[HIV infection and other sexually-transmitted infections among immigrants in Barcelona]', *Enfermedades Infecciosas y Microbiologica Clinica, 20*(4), 154–56.

Wiwanitkit, V., and Waenlor, W. (2002) 'Prevalence of anti-HIV seropositivity in Myanmar migrators in a rural area of Thailand', *Viral Immunology, 15*(4), 661–63.

# Chapter 2

# Leaving loved ones behind

## Mexican gay men's migration to the USA

*Héctor Carrillo*

There is a time in every gay man's life when he has to decide whether to disclose his same-sex attraction to his family. Mexican gay men are no exception. Some choose to disclose and arrive at the decision to *"salir del closet"* (to come out of the closet). Others choose not to disclose and decide instead to fulfill hetero-normative expectations, or at least to pretend to do so. They hide their homosexuality from their families, even in situations where they are aware that their families likely suspect or know that they are not heterosexual. Some even marry women and form families.

Regardless of their decision, however, because Mexican gay men often live in social environments that they perceive to be hostile toward homosexuality, they implement complicated strategies to manage their sexuality to protect themselves and their families from social stigma. Especially among those who choose not to disclose, such management of their sexuality can require vigilance in order to prevent any information about their sexual orientation from reaching their families. Under such circumstances, some men decide to leave Mexico to put some distance between their families and their places of origin. By this route, they seek to reduce the potential for stigma or involuntary disclosure and to be free from the pressures implied in living double lives. They do so also imagining that by moving to the USA they may be able to live freer sexual lives involving sex with other men.

In this chapter, I focus on the intertwined sexual and family-related motivations for migration that Mexican gay and bisexual men report in describing their decisions to leave Mexico and relocate to the USA. Based on ethnographic accounts collected as part of the *Trayectos*[1] study, I analyze how sexual migration is prompted by the structural conditions that surround the enactment of gay identities or, more generally speaking, homoerotic sexual lives in Mexico. For the purposes of this work, I utilize the term *sexual migration* to refer to transnational relocation that is motivated, fully or partially, by the sexualities of those who migrate (Carrillo 2004). From among the list of sexuality-related motivations for migration that Mexican gay and bisexual men recount, I focus in particular on their use of international migration as a strategy to achieve two interrelated purposes: (1) to pursue a kind of sexual liberalization that they imagine is more possible in US cities than within Mexico; and (2) to avoid creating negative situations in the context of their biological family life in Mexico, as well as within their families' social circles, due to their enacting sexual and romantic lives with other men.

The results that I present here contrast greatly with the common finding in survey studies of Mexican migration that the primary motivation for migration is economic. In the cases focused upon, economic motivations are not absent, but they often are not primary. Instead, they linger in the background and appear to be complementary—an added bonus that accompanies the pursuit of other goals. In this sense, this case study demonstrates the importance of considering the multiple motivations for migration that are important for particular population groups who, at the same time that they seek to improve their economic status, are also attempting to find new forms of freedom and to leave behind social conditions that they find oppressive.[2] Thus, my emphasis in the present analysis is not meant to negate or minimize the economic aspects of gay Mexicans' migration to the USA, but rather to highlight concerns and desires that are central and important to them and that are rarely considered in the Mexican migration literature. By focusing on sexual and family-related pressures for migration, my goal is also to highlight the role that sexuality plays in triggering the migration of some Mexicans. As we will see, factors related to social problems such as homophobia and the social stigma of homosexuality not only propel Mexican gay and bisexual men to uproot themselves and leave their places of origin and force them to initiate new lives in places that are often very unfamiliar to them, but also affect their sexual health and create new challenges for them in terms of HIV risk.

## Why leave? Structural violence and social change

Why would Mexican gay and bisexual men wish to leave Mexico due to their sexual orientation? A fairly simple (perhaps simplistic) explanation, and one that commonly circulates in both the USA and in Mexico, including among men in *Trayectos*, is based on the notion that homosexuality is not accepted in Mexico and thus that Mexican gay men are forced to leave because they cannot adopt and enact gay identities or lifestyles in their home country. Among those who take this view, Mexico typically is portrayed as traditional, culturally static, and trapped in the mindset of machismo, while the USA is seen as modern, liberal, and enlightened, particularly in relation to the pursuit of individual rights and the rights of lesbian, gay, bisexual and transgender (LGBT) people. Not only do such depictions present a romanticized view of freedoms in the USA, but they also stand in contrast to the findings from recent sexuality-related research conducted in Mexico. This body of research demonstrates that Mexico has seen considerable social change in relation to sexuality and homosexuality in recent times, particularly over the past three decades (Gutmann 1996; Amuchástegui 2001; Carrillo 2002; González-López 2005; List Reyes 2005), and that since the 1980s the acceptance and visibility of male homosexuality in Mexico has accelerated considerably (Carrillo 2002, 2007; List Reyes 2005).

In Mexico, notions of machismo and male dominance still have cultural valence, but machismo also has been strongly contested, particularly among younger generations. For many Mexicans, the term represents now a past that must be left behind, a label with which one as an individual would never want to be identified (Carrillo 2002; González-López 2005; Gutmann 2007). And, among Mexicans who desire and are actively pursuing sexuality-related personal and social change, a shift in attitudes about homosexuality (at least about male homosexuality) seems also to be happening.

In this regard, Mexico seems to be little different from other countries where an uneven process of change toward increasingly progressive attitudes about sexuality and gender is occurring, perhaps including countries such as the USA. And not unlike other countries, contemporary Mexican sexual cultures are full of what at first glance would appear to be contradictions. But what seems contradictory might instead represent something else. In my research both in Mexico and with immigrant populations, I have identified a fairly seamless co-existence of so-called traditional and modern sexual ideologies, meanings, and cultural practices. Utilizing the concept of cultural hybridity (García-Canclini 1995), I have labeled such co-existence as sexual hybridity and have argued that sexual hybridity allows individual people to make sense of systems of interpretation that at first glance would appear to be contradictory because of the differing meanings that they assign to the same sexual practices. This co-existence of notions of sexual tradition and modernity is of course not unique to Mexico, as work by scholars in other countries has demonstrated (Parker 1991, 1999; Fernández-Alemany and Murray 2002; Sívori 2004; Boellstorff 2005; Padilla 2007).

I do not mean to suggest, however, that sexualities are all the same in all places. Without discounting the role of increasingly global sexualities (Altman 2001), I am also a proponent of the notion that local history and culture play a role in creating differences among countries. Clearly there are differences between Mexico and the USA, both historically and culturally, in terms of the formation of collective gay identities, the strategies that LGBT people utilize to manage their sexualities, and the timing of various political moments in the pursuit of LGBT rights. But it also seems clear that in both countries considerable portions of their respective populations oppose LGBT rights and visibility, while growing segments of their citizenry are in favor of greater sexual equality between heterosexual and homosexual people. Finally, there is evidence that recent events in Mexico in relation to LGBT rights are comparable to those taking place in richer countries, including the USA, and that some may even surpass in scope those that would be possible in this latter context. Examples are the recent approval of civil unions (*sociedades de convivencia*) in Mexico City and the implementation of a national anti-homophobia campaign sponsored by the Mexican federal government (Carrillo 2007; Carrillo and Bliss 2007). The latter in particular would have been inconceivable in the recent political environment in the USA.

In reality, there has not been any study that systematically compares the sexual cultures or sexuality-related historical developments in Mexico and the USA. In other words, the idea that Mexico is more conservative in relation to sexuality and homosexuality than the USA – and that the USA is thus more enlightened than Mexico – rests mainly on a series of assumptions and cultural stereotypes. And, clearly, most gay and bisexually identified men choose to stay and enact their same-sex sexual lives in Mexico where, in spite of any limitations, their situations are constantly improving. So, why then do some Mexican gay men choose to migrate to the USA due to sexual reasons?

In the sections that follow, I provide a preliminary answer to this question by focusing on a combination of immigrants' imaginaries about the sexual liberalism of the USA and their desire to be away from their families of origin in order to enact same-sex sexualities more freely. My analysis rests in part on the concept of structural violence, which proves helpful in understanding the strategies that Mexican gay and bisexual immigrant men use within Mexico to manage their sexualities, as well as how those strategies eventually contribute to their desire to migrate.

Structural violence has been defined in terms of "institutionalized poverty, racism, ethnic discrimination, gender oppression, sexual stigma and oppression, age differentials, and related forms of social inequality" (Parker 2007: 973). In the case that I analyze here, the term is helpful to understand the effects of homophobia, both at the social level and at the level of the social networks in which individuals are immersed: within their immediate and extended families, in their schools and places of work, and in their neighborhoods and towns. For the purposes of this chapter, I think of homophobia as providing the cultural scaffolding that allows people, or even pushes people, to reject gay, lesbian, and bisexual people merely because they are not heterosexual – a rejection that is justified by a generalized perception that it is socially acceptable to dislike homosexuals because of their difference.[3] As we will see, fear of the effects of homophobia, as conceived within the conceptual framework of structural violence, plays an important role in propelling migration for some Mexican gay and bisexual migrants. Before turning to the empirical data, however, I include here a brief description of the study and its methodology.

## The *Trayectos* study

My team and I collected data for this analysis as part of a large ethnographic study of sexuality and HIV risk among gay and bisexual Mexican immigrant men in San Diego, California.[4] *Trayectos* consists of participant observation in places in San Diego where Mexican gay and bisexual immigrant men socialize, and individual in-depth interviews with 150 men. Our interview sample includes Mexican immigrants, US-born Latino men (for comparison), and USA-born sexual/romantic partners of Mexican/Latino men of any race or ethnicity. After an initial in-depth interview, participants were asked to return for a follow-up interview a year later.[5]

A total of 80 men in the study had been raised and socialized in Mexico, all of them of Mexican origin.[6] My discussion here is based primarily on analysis on the interview transcripts of 31 among these 80 men who, in discussing their motivations for migration to the USA, mentioned reasons related to their families of origin or their family life, often combined with reasons related to a desire for greater sexual freedom. Twenty-two of these men were HIV negative, eight were HIV positive, and one had never been tested for HIV. Roughly half of them had engaged in unprotected sexual encounters in the previous year that carried risk for HIV transmission.[7] For the purposes of this analysis, I conducted searches of our coded interview transcripts using codes related to motivations for migration and family. I also examined the narratives on HIV risk for each case.

## Managing disclosure, protecting one's family

> At age 16 I came to live in San Diego, due to economic and family problems, and mainly because of my sexual orientation. I felt a lot of pressure and I was very fearful that my family would find out and that I would start having problems because of that.[8]

These are the words of Aldo,[9] a 32-year-old Mexican man who decided to move to San Diego for the first time when he was 16 years old. Having been born in the border city of Tijuana, Aldo's working-class family had moved around the country while he was growing up, and as a result he had lived as a child in various Mexican cities. Eventually the family settled in Ensenada, approximately 60 miles south of San Diego.

Aldo describes being an effeminate boy and says that other boys teased him for his demeanor and called him *maricón*, a derogatory word in Spanish for effeminate men who are also assumed to engage in homosexual behavior. But he was also good in sports and was a strong child, which somehow compensated for his image as effeminate. Aldo feels that when he was an adolescent, people gossiped behind his back. As he began to realize his sexual attraction to men, he became extremely vigilant about hiding it from others, especially because he had assimilated an extremely negative perception about the meaning of being gay. "The idea that I had of being gay was cruel. I felt like I was worse than a murderer or a rapist," Aldo said. He then added, "Ignorant people believe that gays are incestuous, that we abuse children or want to have sex with everyone, that we are sick ... sexual addicts." When asked how he had acquired those ideas, Aldo referred to his family, which he describes as *homofóbica*. His siblings had contributed to his sense of personal shame by frequently calling him *joto* (another derogatory word for effeminate and homosexual men commonly used in Mexico), which Aldo said was very painful.

Aldo had begun engaging in sexual touching with other boys at age 7 in the context of childhood games, and at age 12 he was anally penetrated in an empty lot by a 27-year-old man he met in the street. Aldo describes being very aroused during the encounter, which led to repeat sexual encounters with this same man when they ran into each other. He also became infatuated with this man. At the same time, however, he wanted to believe this was only a phase that he would grow out of, and that later he would fall in love with a woman, marry her, and have children. This apparent contradiction, which is common, reflected the degree to which Aldo had assimilated heteronormative expectations.

At age 16, Aldo started to go to San Diego on his own using his Mexican passport and US tourist visa. His family was having considerable economic problems, and it was not hard for him to justify to them crossing the border in search of a day job to bring some money back. While in San Diego, he discovered that he could meet men to have sex in the streets, in Balboa Park, and in downtown porn theaters (due to his age he was not allowed into gay bars, dance clubs, or bathhouses).[10] Around the same time, his brother took him to be "sexually initiated" with a female prostitute in Ensenada. His lukewarm response to her confirmed for him that his primary sexual interest was in men.

Aldo was also becoming fearful that his family might find out that he was having sex with men (he described Ensenada as a small town where everyone gossips), and he was also concerned about a situation that had emerged with a rich, professional man in Ensenada he had dated when he was 15 years old. Angry after this man dismissed him and stopped giving him money, Aldo had threatened the man by telling him he would report him to the police for sexual abuse; the man in return had asked another person, who claimed to be a policeman, to threaten Aldo.

It was at that point that Aldo decided to move, at least part time, to California. San Diego rapidly became a place where he could escape the pressure that he felt while being in Ensenada. The first time that he traveled to San Diego he had met a Mexican man with whom he had sex, but who also helped him find work in a restaurant. Aldo initiated a pattern of enacting his gay sexuality in San Diego, and then comfortably returning to Ensenada to enact his family life without concern about being found out by his parents and siblings. Not unlike other Mexican gay and bisexual immigrant men, Aldo used the distance from his family as a management strategy that allowed him to avoid the pressure that he felt from his parents and siblings and that also reduced the need for him to disclose his sexual orientation to them.[11] At age 28 he decided to move permanently to San Diego.

When he was interviewed for *Trayectos*, Aldo had not disclosed his homosexuality to his family. But he also said that in his family his sexual orientation is a "*secreto a voces*," an open secret. In describing the sense that his family must know that he is gay, he used the phrase "*lo que se ve no se pregunta*" ("why ask about what can simply be seen"), famously employed in a television interview some years before by the Mexican singer Juan Gabriel when avoiding a direct response to a reporter's question about whether he was gay.

In talking about his family, Aldo mostly seemed concerned about their not finding out openly that he is gay, in order to protect himself from their possible negative reaction. Other immigrant men, however, emphasize instead that their migration was motivated by a desire to protect their families from social stigma. For instance Humberto, age 29, grew up in a small town in the Mexican southern state of Guerrero. When he was a child, Humberto's father believed strongly in a strictly gendered distribution of masculine and feminine tasks:

> My father would tell us that if we swept the floors, cooked, cleaned the dishes, or made the beds, if we did feminine tasks ... that those things were for women. He would be unforgiving about seeing us do such things; he would hit us and mistreat us. On the other hand, I would see my uncles who would ask my male cousins to sweep, cook, and nothing [bad] happened, and my uncles were all men.

Humberto's father would tell him and his brothers that if they turned out to be *jotos*, he would throw them out. Humberto feels that his father's behavior severely traumatized him, and for that reason he later ended up despising his father. But he loved his mother, who he found caring and understanding.

By age 15, Humberto fully knew that he was sexually attracted to men. Earlier, a young man who was living with his grandparents had forced him to have sex. At age 17, he began to make out with women, but he never had sex with one. And by age 18 he consciously began to pursue sex with male friends his own age in the context of friendship – sex that often took place after soccer or basketball matches. Humberto was concerned, however, that in his small town word could spread about the fact that he had sex with men, and that as a result his family would suffer social stigma.

Humberto knew that his father did not have money to pay for him to attend college. After he lost his job, through her connections his mother helped him obtain a new job in a Tijuana factory. He had a friend who had moved to San Diego, and this man encouraged him to cross the border, which he did just two weeks after arriving in Tijuana. Humberto joined two others who crossed over the hills into the USA without documents. In talking about his decision to leave his home town and to not only move to Tijuana but also to cross into San Diego, Humberto said: "I wanted to get out of there. I wanted to be far from my family ... to not harm them emotionally. Do you understand? That people would start talking, 'your son is like that.'" Humberto's narrative suggests, however, that his family itself also had already become a source of pressure:

> I wanted to leave due to my family, because they harassed me, they could see what I was doing. ... I wanted to leave because I didn't want to con- tinue acting [as they expected me to act]. I already knew my situation; I knew that I was gay and that I liked men.

Humberto thus felt that his departure would both protect his family from social stigma and reduce the pressure for him so that he could live a freer life.

For gay men such as Humberto and Aldo, the pressure that they felt emanating from their families takes two forms. Families constantly remind them, directly or subtly, of their heteronormative expectations in terms of marriage to a woman, having children, etc. Second, families expect that unmarried children live in the family home, which limits their ability to pursue their sexual lives with other men. Out of respect for their families, they often do not disclose openly their homosexuality, and even when they do, a sense of respect also sometimes prevents them from integrating their own lives into their family life. As Augusto (age 31) put it:

> I was not thinking of going back. I wanted to be independent. In Culiacán I was never going to leave my family home. … That's how Mexican culture is … you live with your parents all the time. It's rare [to leave them] unless you go to study elsewhere. So, I wanted to get out.

For these adult men, living with their families means not being able to have sex at home, or even have the liberty of inviting boyfriends or gay friends to visit them—a complete separation between their family life (where often they are presumed to be heterosexual, despite their families being aware or suspecting that they are not) and their gay life. Moving by themselves to the USA provides welcome distance from their families, and their migrating is easily socially justifiable, particularly because they often end up sending money to their families after migrating. In some cases, however, they do not make the decision to move to the USA alone, and in fact the families of some of them play a central role in promoting their departure.

## Complicit families

In the narratives of several immigrant men in *Trayectos*, their families figure prominently as actors that encouraged them to leave Mexico. As we already saw, Mexican gay immigrants' families benefit from these men's migration to the USA in more ways than one. In addition to financial benefits in situations of economic need, which are very common, the immigrant's absence also translates into several social benefits. The immigrants report that for their families international migration provides an easy way for them to justify to their local social networks why their son or sibling left. Their departure also becomes an antidote against local social stigma, both for the gay or bisexual man and for the family. Moreover, promoting the migration of gay sons reflects a fear on the part of parents that if they stay they may face a difficult life, and also that negative social reactions to their son's homosexuality will affect not only the son, but the family as a whole.

As parents recognize for themselves their son's "difference," they sometimes incrementally build the process leading to a suggestion to migrate. But in some of the cases, migration is also precipitated rather suddenly after specific events take place that trigger immediate family intervention. This is well exemplified by the story of Tadeo, a 28 year old who was born in the USA but who was raised in Guadalajara. When asked why he moved to California, Tadeo responded:

> Because my mother used to tell me since I was a kid that I wasn't meant to be in Mexico. Why? Because society was so rude and it was going to be rude to me when I was starting to go out on the street and go to school, and if I had that problem that … I go out and people … harass me about sexual things and about my personality, then she was going to be sad.

In this account, Tadeo uses the word "personality" as a euphemism for "homosexuality." Noticing that Tadeo was different, his mother had taken a pragmatic approach, in part because the family is very religious and conservative (they regularly attend a Jehovah's Witness church) and she feared that Tadeo would suffer discrimination within the family's social circles. His father also repeatedly encouraged him to move to San Diego, where the parents had personal connections. On one occasion, he even addressed the topic of homosexuality in a generic way, telling Tadeo that being gay did not have to mean losing one's manhood.[12] Apparently, this comment was in reaction to Tadeo's shyness and effeminacy. It is noteworthy that his parents breached this topic even prior to Tadeo's adopting and disclosing a gay identity, as in fact Tadeo acknowledged to himself he is gay only after arriving in the USA.

Tadeo's permanent departure from Mexico was precipitated by a very unfortunate event that took place in his family home. On one occasion when his parents were away, Tadeo arrived home and found one of his older brothers drinking with some of his male friends. They offered him a drink, which he reluctantly accepted. They gave him a beer, which Tadeo took to his room. Some time after drinking the beer, Tadeo felt very sick. He managed to call an ambulance before passing out. He now believes that his brother and his friends had put sleeping pills in his beer. When the paramedics arrived at the house, they found Tadeo's brother and his friends naked in Tadeo's room, where Tadeo was also naked and unconscious. Tadeo later pressed charges for sexual abuse (he was still 17 at the time) and his brother and some of his friends, all of whom were well known within the church that the family attended, ended up going to jail. At that point—and despite the fact that Tadeo was the victim in this encounter—his parents insisted that he had to leave to California.

Another interesting case is that of Justo, a 32 year old from a small city in the Mexican state of Jalisco. When Justo was 19 his father rummaged through his backpack. The father found and read a letter that had been written by a man whom Justo was dating. Justo says that it was very unusual for his father to do this, because in his house there was a strongly stated rule of respect for the privacy of everyone's belongings. My interpretation is that, being already suspicious of his son's homosexuality, Justo's father was unable to ask him directly and instead looked for evidence that would confirm his suspicion.

Justo is grateful, however, that his father read the letter, because his father's reaction facilitated his process of moving to the USA. When Justo came home that day, his father told him that he had read the letter and that he preferred to know. It appears that the father had become suspicious because of people's insinuations that Justo was gay. At that point the father offered to take him to have sex with a woman, so that he could be sure about whether he was truly gay or not. When Justo responded he was not interested, the father told him that he himself had a gay friend and that his friend had suffered enormously during his life. The father also expressed conditional support. As Justo put it:

> He said, "If that's what you want, go ahead. I support you. You will still be my son. *Mijo*, I'll ask you just one thing. If you ever plan to do something that could shame the family, don't do it here. That's the only thing that I ask of you. I don't ask anything else. For me and for your grandfather, because you know that he is well known here." And I said, "Sure, that's fine." That's why I came here. That's why I am here.

Justo interpreted his father's request that he did nothing in his home town that could shame the family—meaning any open enacting of his homosexuality—as a clear appeal for him to leave and be gay somewhere else, where no one in the family's social circles could see it.

Finally, Facundo, age 36, was born in Durango but after his mother died when he was 16, he moved to Tijuana with his siblings to live with an aunt. In Tijuana he had a relationship with a boyfriend that lasted eight years, beginning when he was 21. Without ever disclosing his sexual orientation to his family, he integrated this man into his family life. In doing this Facundo seemed to rely on the management strategy known as sexual silence (Díaz 1998; Carrillo 2002). Everybody in his family appeared to know indirectly that they were boyfriends, but Facundo's sexual orientation or his relationship with this man were never openly discussed. In Facundo's story it is clear that his family accepted the relationship and had also accepted Facundo's boyfriend as part of the extended family. The boyfriend attended all the family events, and the family would ask where he was if he did not show up.

When the couple broke up, Facundo became very depressed and even suicidal, which led him to be hospitalized. Moreover, his now ex-boyfriend was stalking him. Concerned, his family began to ask questions about what had happened, where the boyfriend was, and why he no longer was around. At that point one brother decided to finally broach the topic. Facundo said, "One of my brothers told me: 'Let's speak frankly. I know what it is. Please confirm it.' I told him: 'There's nothing to confirm. Life will continue to be the same, but, yes, I am gay.'" Once disclosure took place, and Facundo was able to tell his siblings and extended family what was happening, a female cousin who lived in San Diego suggested that he cross the border and go live on the US side:

... she tells me: "Come here. He lives in Tijuana. He won't come looking for you here. He will not be able to come harm you." He continued to pursue me, and he was tormenting me. ... My family told me, "You must go to San Diego because you have to create a different life and meet different people, because this thing is hurting you too much."

As these cases illustrate, Mexican gay immigrants' families take action and openly suggest to them that they must leave in situations in which they fear for their safety, are aiming to protect them, or are concerned that the gay man's sexual orientation will generate shame and stigma for the family. In that sense they become complicit in turning their sons and siblings effectively into sexual exiles (or "sexiles," to use the term coined by Manolo Guzmán) who depart from Mexico in order to leave behind difficult personal situations or to preempt them.

## New freedoms, new challenges

In discussing their lives in the USA, immigrant men such as the ones whose stories I have presented here tend to talk about their experiences of migration as indeed creating a respite from the pressures and forms of structural violence that pushed them away from their places of origin. But they also express enormous longing for the things they left behind. Consider the case of Aldo, whom I quoted earlier. A few months after moving for the first time to San Diego, he decided to return to Mexico to live with his family: "So I came to the United States, but I went back soon after, because I was very depressed. I was there about eight months, and then I went back." It took Aldo several years before he could make the decision again to leave, this time for good. For some men like Aldo, their longing for their homes, families, and everything familiar becomes especially acute once they encounter what they perceive as extreme American individualism (and all that accompanies it) and realize that they now miss enormously the collective orientation that characterized their family and social life back home.

Generally speaking, living in the USA, away from their families, does allow these men to explore their sexual lives in a different way than they imagine they could in Mexico, in part because of their encounters with new sexual cultures, and in part simply because now they do not feel that they have someone watching over their shoulders at all times. But the change also brings new challenges related to their sexuality, as I have described in greater detail elsewhere (Carrillo et al. 2008). In the USA their new freedoms often gain men access to sexual contexts that are unfamiliar to them, and which they must learn to navigate without a map (although sometimes other gay immigrants prove to be helpful resources). From learning about the existence of gay neighborhoods in US cities, to encountering institutionalized spaces that facilitate easy casual encounters (such as the gay bathhouses), to realizing that they can lead steady romantic relations openly with a man (which may or may not involve sexual

exclusivity), Mexican gay and bisexual immigrant men find themselves encountering new and exciting possibilities, but also new risks. These challenges that
stem from exposure to new contexts are further compounded by potential mis-
understandings within cross-cultural relations that relate to differing perceptions
about the severity of HIV disease and the responsibility of sexual partners to
protect each other.

Turning specifically to the 31 men included in this analysis, migration had
mixed effects on their sexualities and HIV risk. As mentioned, roughly half had
recently engaged in unprotected sexual intercourse with male partners of opposite or unknown HIV status. For some in the subgroup who had unprotected
sex, these encounters represented an increase in HIV risk after migration. For
others the opposite occurred: in Mexico they had never used condoms, while in
the USA they began to use them sporadically due to increased access to HIV/
AIDS education, except in contexts that were challenging or unfamiliar.

The six men quoted in this chapter—whose cases most eloquently illustrate
the intersection of family- and sexuality related motivations for migration—
encountered new forms of HIV risk in the USA. However, it is interesting to
note that all six of them managed to remain HIV negative. They did so in spite
of the destabilization in their lives and the personal burdens that resulted from
their being alone and away from their home towns. Aldo, for instance, suffered
constant depression and loneliness that he related to being away from familiar
spaces in Mexico (although, paradoxically, he felt also that being freer sexually
in San Diego helped reduce his depression). To lessen his loneliness in San
Diego, he began to attend gay support groups.[13] Simultaneously, he also
engaged in casual sex with a growing number of sexual partners (mostly in gay
bathhouses, which he was not familiar with before moving to San Diego), and he
became quite concerned about what he called "sexual compulsivity." He may
have learned that term in the support groups themselves, or in an Alcoholics
Anonymous group that he attended after he began worrying about the large
amount of alcohol he was drinking.

Although he tried to look for a steady partner with whom he could share his
life, Aldo had difficulties finding the right boyfriend. In the context of his life in
San Diego, however, Aldo managed to use condoms consistently. He connected
his ability to use condoms to a strong fear of HIV, which served him as a constant reminder of the need to stay safe, including in sexual situations in which
other immigrant men like him were unable to use condoms. At the time of his
follow-up interview (a year after the initial one), he had moved to Tijuana, but he
crossed the border daily for work. He continued to have sex in gay bathhouses in
San Diego, and he now also had sex with men in Tijuana porn theaters.

For Humberto, sexual freedom while living away from his family has taken a
very different meaning. Coming from a small town in Mexico where sexual
relations between men were heavily gendered, Humberto despised the idea of
frequenting dance clubs full of gay men or having gay men as sexual partners. In
San Diego he replicated the same patterns of sexual interaction that he knew in

his home town. He mostly had sex with heterosexually identified, married, Mexican immigrant men, and he let his sexual partners decide whether to use a condom or not. However, in one unprotected sexual encounter that Humberto described in detail, his partner withdrew before ejaculating as a risk reduction strategy. When we interviewed Humberto again a year after his initial interview, he reported having found out that a friend had tested positive for HIV, and this made him decide to become more cautious about his own HIV risk.

The other four men whom I quoted had found new forms of sex in San Diego that were also context specific. They shared a desire for maintaining long-term relationships with a man. Augusto had accessed networks of gay men who used crystal methamphetamine, and he had a recent history of relationships with men from those networks with whom he sometimes did not use condoms (one later confessed having unprotected sex with an HIV-positive man while dating Augusto). Justo's partner of five years made the decision for them to discard condoms after a year into their relationship. Justo suspected that his partner was unfaithful, which concerned him. Facundo strongly emphasized condom use, but he did not use them with a steady partner who later confessed being unfaithful. Facundo reported difficulties asking Latino men to use condoms and said that with those men a condom can "ruin the moment." In his opinion, white American men have more of a "culture of condoms." Yet, aside from his experiences with the steady partner, Facundo managed to use condoms consistently, and so did Tadeo, who initiated his sexual life with men only after arriving in the USA. In general terms, the fact that several among these six men recently had found themselves in situations that involved risk demonstrated that their ability to use protection in San Diego was somewhat fragile.

## Conclusion

As the cases discussed here illustrate, sexual and family-related motivations play an important role in Mexican gay and bisexual men's migration to the USA. Their departure makes things better for all, at least on the surface: it relieves the heteronormative pressures that the families exert, reduces the potential for gay men and their families to experience negative social reactions, and opens up spaces for the gay men to live their sexualities more openly while away from their families. Ironically, these men's departure may also prevent the immigrants and their families from addressing the underlying factors—the negative effects of structural violence that in part made the immigrants leave in the first place.

In connection to these immigrant men's sexual health and HIV risk, the role that leaving their families plays is somewhat unclear. On the one hand, for some of these men the change is dramatic in terms of their sense of loneliness and isolation. They lose access to tight kinship networks in which they previously lived all their lives. Some have rough encounters with American individualism, and as a result experience isolation and even depression. These are factors that the psychological literature often connects with heightened HIV risk (Díaz 1998).

On the other hand, distance from family also promotes greater independence and sexual freedom, which several of these men appreciate. And some manage well the challenge of entering new sexual contexts, while others do not.

These men's families may hope that by leaving Mexico the immigrants will have a better life in the USA, but the conditions under which they leave can end up preventing their families from helping them prepare to confront the mental and sexual health risks that they may encounter after relocation. It remains unclear whether Mexican gay and bisexual immigrant men can achieve what they wish for by migrating while simultaneously maintaining their family's support and renewing their relationship with their families in a way that fits whoever they become in the USA. In relation to their sexual risk for HIV, a key research and policy question is what can be done to ensure that the immigrants' journey translates not into peril rather but into an opportunity to live a healthier sexual life—one that includes support from the families who saw them leave.

## Notes

1 *Trayectos* is a Spanish word that means trajectory or path.
2 In relation to gender, see studies conducted with Mexican women, which identify gender- and sexuality related motivations for migration, including desires to leave behind expectations of sexual modesty and the desire to redefine relationships in a more egalitarian manner (Hondagneu-Sotelo 1994; González-López 2005; Hirsch 2003). See also work with Mexican gay and bisexual migrants by Lionel Cantú (2001).
3 According to Savin-Williams (2001:15) "homonegativity" may be a more accurate term to describe situations in which homosexuality is seen as "not an equally viable way of life" compared to heterosexuality. I have chosen to use the term "homophobia" because it denotes a full range of negative attitudes toward homosexuality, all of which contribute to widespread structural violence (even if indirect and not verbal or physical) toward LGBT people.
4 The *Trayectos* Study is supported by Award Number R01HD042919 from the US National Institute of Child Health and Human Development. The content is solely the responsibility of the authors and does not necessarily represent the official views of the National Institute of Child Health and Human Development or the National Institutes of Health.
5 Our interviews were conducted in Spanish or English, according to the participants' preferences. Of the original sample of 150 men, 115 (77 percent) returned for a follow-up interview. All interviews were audio-recorded, transcribed verbatim and coded. The resulting coded transcripts were entered into QSR N6.0, a software package for the management and systematic analysis of qualitative data.
6 Five in this subsample were born in the USA but lived in Mexico in their childhood. In terms of sexual socialization, their experiences are not considerably different from those who were born in Mexico.
7 Here I define HIV risk as unprotected anal intercourse with partners of opposite or unknown HIV status. Participants were asked to provide detailed accounts of such encounters that took place within the previous year. An important clarification is that in some of those encounters the insertive partner withdrew before ejaculation
8 I have translated into English quotations from interviews that were originally conducted in Spanish.
9 The names of all study participants are pseudonyms.

10  In the interview, it is unclear how he managed to be allowed into porn theaters.
11  Many participants in this study did not want to distance themselves from their families, but saw it as a necessity to hide their homosexuality from them. Some however, wanted distance from their families to avoid the extreme pressures that the families exerted upon them.
12  Tadeo feels that his late father may have been bisexual.
13  As also found by Cantú (2001), upon arrival in the USA Mexican gay immigrants seek and find support within gay networks, or what Kath Weston calls "chosen families."

## References

Altman, D. (2001) *Global Sex*, Chicago and London: University of Chicago Press.

Amuchástegui, A. (2001) *Virginidad e iniciación sexual en México: Experiencias y significados*, Mexico City: Edamex.

Boellstorff, T. (2005) *The Gay Archipelago: Sexuality and Nation in Indonesia*, Princeton: Princeton University Press.

Cantú, L. (2001) 'A Place Called Home: A Queer Political Economy of Mexican Immigrant Men's Family Experiences', in M. Bernstein and R. Reimann (eds) *Queer Families, Queer Politics: Challenging Culture and the State*, New York: Columbia University Press.

Carrillo, H. (2002) *The Night is Young: Sexuality in Mexico in the Time of AIDS*, Chicago and London: University of Chicago Press.

——(2004) 'Sexual Migration, Cross-Cultural Sexual Encounters, and Sexual Health', *Sexuality Research & Social Policy*, 1(3): 58–70.

——(2007) 'Imagining Modernity: Sexuality, Policy, and Social Change in Mexico', *Sexuality, Research & Social Policy*, 4(3): 74–91.

Carrillo, H. and Bliss, K. (2007) 'Introduction to Special Issue. Nuevas Direcciones: Sexuality, Politics, and Reproductive Health in Mexico', *Sexuality, Research & Social Policy*, 4(3): 1–5.

Carrillo, H., Fontdevila, J., Brown, J. and Gómez, W. (2008) *Risk Across Borders. Sexual Contexts and HIV Prevention Challenges among Mexican Gay and Bisexual Immigrant Men. Findings and Recommendations from the* Trayectos *Study*. Online. Available from: www.caps.ucsf. edu/projects/Trayectos/monograph/EnglishFinal.pdf (accessed August 8, 2008).

Díaz, R. M. (1998) *Latino Gay Men and HIV*, New York: Routledge.

Fernández-Alemany, M. and Murray, S. O. (2002) *Heterogender Homosexuality in Honduras*, San Jose: Writers Club Press.

García-Canclini, N. (1995) *Hybrid Cultures: Strategies for Entering and Leaving Modernity*, Minneapolis: University of Minnesota Press.

González-López, G. (2005) *Erotic Journeys: Mexican Immigrants and their Sex Lives*, Berkeley: University of California Press.

Gutmann, M. (1996) *The Meanings of Macho: Being a Man in Mexico City*, Berkeley: University of California Press.

——(2007) *Fixing Men: Sex, Birth Control, and AIDS in Mexico*, Berkeley: University of California Press.

Hirsch, J. S. (2003) *A Courtship after Marriage: Sexuality and Love in Mexican Transnational Families*, Berkeley, Los Angeles, and London: University of California Press.

Hondagneu-Sotelo, P. (1994) *Gendered Transitions: Mexican Experiences of Immigration*, Berkeley: University of California Press.

List Reyes, M. (2005) *Jóvenes Corazones Gay en la Ciudad de México*, Puebla: Benemérica Universidad Autónoma de Puebla.

Padilla, M. B. (2007) *Caribbean Pleasure Industry: Tourism, Sexuality, and AIDS in the Dominican Republic*, Chicago and London: University of Chicago Press.

Parker, R. (1991) *Bodies, Pleasures, and Passions: Sexual Culture in Contemporary Brazil*, Boston: Beacon Press.

——(1999) *Beneath the Equator: Cultures of Desire, Male Homosexuality, and Emerging Gay Communities in Brazil*, New York: Routledge.

——(2007) 'Sexuality, Health, and Human Rights', *American Journal of Public Health*, 97(6): 972–73.

Savin-Williams, R. C. (2001) *Mom, Dad. I'm Gay: How Families Negotiate Coming Out*, Washington, DC: American Psychological Association.

Sívori, H. F. (2004) *Locas, chongos y gays: Sociabilidad homosexual masculina durante la década de 1990*, Buenos Aires: Antropofagia.

# Chapter 3

# Concentrated disadvantages

## Neighbourhood context as a structural risk for Latino immigrants in the USA

*Emilio A. Parrado, Chenoa A. Flippen and Leonardo Uribe*

Understanding how context relates to risk behaviours has been a central concern in social science and public health research. The issue is especially salient in migration studies since migration by definition entails an often dramatic change in context that can have a profound impact on well-being. Despite its significance, research connecting migration and HIV has often overlooked the relationship between context and risk behaviours. The bulk of HIV research tends to follow individualistic behavioural models (Organista *et al.* 2004) which cannot account for the considerable variation in risk behaviours according to where migrants reside. As such, the social mechanisms mediating the association between migration and HIV remain unclear.

In this study we follow a contextual approach to HIV risk among Latino migrants to the USA, examining the neighbourhood context of reception and its connection with the concentration of risks. Building on classical and contemporary social disorganization theory we show that immigrants' exposure to HIV risk does not occur in a vacuum but rather concentrates across well-defined neighbourhoods in conjunction with other health risks and structural disadvantages.

The empirical analysis combines quantitative and qualitative information collected across 32 Latino migrants receiving neighbourhoods in Durham/Carrboro, North Carolina. The analytic strategy is to describe the considerable variation in neighbourhood contexts of reception and their association with health risks. Results show that macro-level forces associated with immigration policies and the structural position of Latino populations in the USA undergird much of immigrants' exposure to health risks, and that identifying the neighbourhoods' concentrating disadvantages can be particularly instrumental for more localized and cost-effective interventions aimed at reducing HIV transmission among migrants.

## Neighbourhoods and migrant health risks

The connection between context and behaviour has been a classical concern in the immigrant adaptation literature; migration entails not only a shift in residence but also a process of social change resulting from exposure to different behaviours, norms, and people. Early studies of immigrant adaptation centred on identifying behavioural changes associated with differences between countries of origin and destination. In their classic study of Polish peasants relocating in Europe and America, Thomas and Znaniecki (1920) described the process as a socially disorganizing experience. Migrants leave behind structures of social support and control emanating from long-term friendship and family networks. At destination, the weaker structures of social support and control limit migrants' ability to deal with their new environment, encouraging problems of crime, family violence, and depression. Thus, contextual processes resulting from differential community structures directly connected with behavioural outcomes.

While classical social disorganization theory framed these negative effects as an almost universal consequence of migration, subsequent research shows that migration can also be a liberating experience enhancing immigrants' personal development (Brody 1970). Moreover, there is considerable variation in adaptation reflecting personal socioeconomic and demographic characteristics emanating from the context of exit, such as age, gender, and occupation (Alba and Nee 2003). Adaptation also varies according to broader dimensions of the context of reception, such as labour market conditions, immigration policies, and the size of the co-ethnic community (Portes and Rumbaut 2006). Attention to the contexts of origin and reception has been instrumental for understanding variation in the pace of adaptation across national-origin groups. However, the interactional processes accounting for *within*-group variation in outcomes remain under-explored.

To understand the interactional processes connecting context and risk among immigrants we have sought to apply theoretical developments in social disorganization theory from the criminological literature. Based on the observation that neighbourhood patterns of deviance tend to remain constant over time in spite of continuous population change, criminologists argue that crime is not exclusively an individual-level phenomenon but rather correlates with the ecological environment in which it occurs (Shaw and McKay 1942). In this framework, social disorganization is defined as the inability of communities to realize the common values of their residents and maintain effective social control; a major dimension of which is the supervision and control of young, single men. The local community comprises a system of formal and informal friendship, kinship and acquaintanceship networks (Sampson 1988); variation in this social control-producing system is thus central to neighbourhood differences in deviance.

Three elements from criminological perspectives on social disorganization are instrumental for understanding risk behaviours among contemporary immigrants. The first is the recognition of the *spatial concentration* of risks. Rather than being randomly distributed across metropolitan areas, risk behaviours tend to cluster in neighbourhoods that show remarkable stability over time and become an avenue of risk exposure for new residents. The second is that high rates of deviance overlap with other *structural disadvantages*, particularly poverty, ethnic heterogeneity, and population turnover. These structural conditions can contribute to social deviance (including some sexual risk behaviours) by undermining the interactional and institutional processes that generate social control. And finally, *gender composition* represents an additional structural disadvantage of migrant neighbourhoods. Building on feminist theory, Hagan and colleagues formulated a power-control theory of deviance that stresses the role of women as instruments and objects of informal social control (Hagan *et al.* 1987). Role differentiation in patriarchal societies renders women more involved in social control and affectionate care than men, assigning them a moral prominence and guardians of 'decent' behaviours. Migration, especially in the Latin American–USA context, significantly affects the gender composition of communities. Family separation and the over-representation of single men reduce the presence of women in receiving communities, which both limits the dating market for Latino men and undermines the social control function provided by women's influence.

## Setting and analytical strategy

We investigate the spatial distribution of risks and their association with structural disadvantages among Latino immigrants in Durham, North Carolina. Part of the larger trend of the dispersion of the Latino population, migrants were drawn to the area in the 1990s in response to the high tech boom in the nearby research triangle and the concomitant demand for workers in construction and service industries. In response, the Latino population (roughly 70 per cent from Mexico and the remainder primarily from Honduras, Guatemala, and El Salvador) experienced rapid growth, increasing from less than 1 to 9 per cent of the total population between 1990 and 2000. The relatively recent arrival of Latino migrants is evident in data from the 2000 Census, which shows that nearly 75 per cent are born outside the USA, with more than 85 per cent arriving after 1990. Not surprisingly, the vast majority is undocumented, exhibit relatively low levels of English fluency, and are concentrated in low-skill employment.

Like many areas of new migrant destination, the gender composition of the Latino population is highly uneven. While Latina women increasingly participate in migration to the USA, the difficulties, danger, and expense associated with border crossing, especially with young children, discourage the migration of both single and married women. In Durham, the effects are dramatic as there are more than two men aged 20–29 for every woman in the same age range. As a result, areas of high Latino concentration have become targets for a well-developed sex industry, which includes nearby street-walking sex workers, a number of brothels, and groups of women who visit the apartments themselves, soliciting men gathered in common areas or searching out former clients. In addition, a small number of bars and clubs tailored to serve the Latino community provide night time recreational activities. While women in these bars are less numerous than men, they include both Latinas and Anglo women, providing an avenue for non-commercial social interactions and access to the wider dating market.

The relatively recent development of the Durham Latino community required special considerations to approximate a representative sample. Our study relied heavily on Community Based Participatory Research (CBPR), which uses a critical theoretical perspective which includes the 'local theory' of community participants as collaborators in the research process (Parrado et al. 2005). In our case, a group of 20 Latino men and women from the community were directly involved in every stage of the research, including formulation of the questionnaire, identification of survey locales, and lending culturally grounded interpretation to the analyses. In addition, the CBPR group was trained in survey methods and conducted all interviews, enhancing data quality and helping achieve a refusal rate of 10.7 per cent.

We also employed targeted random sampling. Specifically, we conducted a census of all housing units in 35 apartment complexes/blocks and 13 trailer parks that house large numbers of migrant Latinos. Using this as our sampling frame, we randomly selected individual units to be visited by interviewers, culminating in 1,522 face-to-face interviews with migrant Latino men aged 18 to 49.

One advantage of the targeted design is that the selected areas of Latino concentration closely approximate theoretical conceptualization of neighbourhoods (rather than administrative units like census tracts). Thus, our sampling units represent spatially identifiable environments separate from the larger context. In addition, the sampling units function as the area of residence where people spend most of their free time, develop friendships, get together to play cards or drink, and recreate during the weekend. It is this spatial and interactional configuration that also serves to concentrate HIV risk factors.

For the current analysis we limit our sample to men, who engage in more risk behaviours than women and to the 32 neighbourhoods where at least 10 migrant Latino men were interviewed. We use the individual-level data to construct aggregate measures of health risks and indicators of social disorganization and employ data from our sampling frame to measure neighbourhood ethnic composition.

## Results

### Neighbourhood variation in health risks and social disorganization

Table 3.1 reports descriptive statistics of health risk and social disorganization indicators. The two main sources of HIV risk in the Durham Latino community are sex with commercial and casual partners. We collected data on drug use and the use of syringes, including needle sharing. The former was relatively uncommon and the latter virtually non-existent among local migrants. In addition, less than 1.5 per cent of respondents reported sexual experience with other men.

*Table 3.1* Neighbourhood variation in health risks and social disorganization among Latino men

|  | Mean | SD | Min | Max |
|---|---|---|---|---|
| *Health and sexual risks* | | | | |
| Use of sex worker (%) | 22.7 | 11.3 | 0.0 | 45.9 |
| Casual partner (%) | 23.8 | 9.5 | 5.6 | 44.4 |
| Heavy drinker (%)[a] | 26.2 | 11.7 | 0.0 | 55.6 |
| Feelings of depression (mean)[b] | 4.7 | 0.5 | 3.8 | 6.3 |
| *Social disorganization* | | | | |
| Median wages | 9.9 | 1.0 | 8.0 | 12.3 |
| Recent arrival (%) | 45.4 | 12.0 | 23.1 | 75.0 |
| Non-Hispanic residents (%) | 20.5 | 12.7 | 2.1 | 42.5 |
| *Gender-related migration dynamics* | | | | |
| Unaccompanied men (%) | 60.8 | 13.7 | 27.6 | 84.2 |
| Appartments with female resident (%) | 61.0 | 15.6 | 31.6 | 94.4 |
| N | 32 | | | |

[a]Heavy drinkers were defined as those who reported four or more drinks, three or more times per week, or those consuming more than six drinks on any one day.
[b]Mental health problems were assessed using the 10-item CES-D screening for depression. The dichotomous agree/disagree format of the scale is particularly well suited for the relatively low educational level of recent Latino immigrants and has been found to work well among the population (Robison *et al.* 2002). A cut-off point of 3 or 4 has been suggested for identifying depression. However, for our purposes a continuous measure agreement with depressive statements provides more detailed information about variation in outcomes.

However, estimates show that nearly one-quarter of all men reported a commercial sex partner in the previous year; among both single and unaccompanied married men the figure was nearly 40 per cent. Commercial sex can be a source of HIV, because it acts as a potential bridge between high-risk and low-risk populations, both through inconsistent condom use and because of the higher number of partners implied. While roughly 90 per cent of men reported using condoms with sex workers, only 64 per cent reported they would use a condom if the sex worker were known to them (Parrado *et al.* 2004).

An additional 23 per cent of men reported a casual sexual partner in the previous year, including 41 per cent of single men and 22 per cent of unaccompanied married men. Casual partners are also a potential source of HIV; only 70 per cent of men report using condoms with casual partners, far lower than the figure for commercial sex, and a full 22 per cent of unaccompanied married men report never using condoms with their casual partners. Moreover, there is dramatic variation across neighbourhoods in the incidence of risk behaviours; in some settings literally no men report commercial and casual partners while in others nearly half do so. Other health risks, namely excessive alcohol consumption and depression, also vary across neighbourhoods, particularly the former. For instance, while the average rate of heavy drinking is 26 per cent, neighbourhood rates vary from essentially zero to nearly 56 per cent.

Elements of social disorganization also vary considerably across neighbourhoods. In addition to modest neighbourhood differences in average wages, the concentration of recently arrived immigrants varies widely. While 45 per cent of Latinos have been in the area for less than three years their representation ranges from 23 to 75 per cent. Recent arrivals, possibly because they are less well connected to other avenues for social support and emotional expression, are more likely than their better established counterparts to visit sex workers. Likewise, on average, Latino immigrants reside in neighbourhoods that are only 21 per cent non-Latino. However, the range extends from areas almost completely Latino (98 per cent) to areas that are 43 per cent non-Latino.

Gender composition also varies dramatically across neighbourhoods. Nearly 61 per cent of Latino migrant men in Durham are unaccompanied, that is, either single or married to partners who continue to reside in their country of origin. But the concentration of unaccompanied men across neighbourhoods varies from a low of 28 to a high of 84 per cent. Likewise, only 61 per cent of Latino households in Durham contain at least one woman, but in some neighbourhoods as few as 32 per cent do so while in others nearly all apartments (94 per cent) contain women.

### Association between health risks and social disorganization

Pearson correlation coefficients were computed to assess the association between health risks and social disorganization. This was then followed by a common factor analysis to create an index of concentrated disadvantage. This index was used to construct a typology of neighbourhoods according to their degree of risk concentration that we map and describe both quantitatively and qualitatively to further elaborate on the connection between spatial processes and individual risk exposure.

The correlation matrix presented in Table 3.2 shows a clear association among health risk indicators. Commercial sex, casual relationships, and heavy drinking are all positively associated, as are heavy drinking and depression. Health risks, particularly sex worker use, are also correlated with indicators of social disorganization. Neighbourhoods with a higher share of recently arrived immigrants and of unaccompanied men average higher rates of commercial sex. At the other end of the risk spectrum, the share of households that are not Latino or with female residents is negatively associated with neighbourhood-level commercial sex.

The association between other health risks is less consistent. Casual partnerships are significantly more common in neighbourhoods with a higher share of unaccompanied men and less common in areas with greater female

Table 3.2 Correlation matrix and factor loadings among neighbourhood indicators of risk

| | (1) | (2) | (3) | (4) | (5) | (6) | (7) | (8) | (9) | Factor loadings |
|---|---|---|---|---|---|---|---|---|---|---|
| (1) Use of sex worker (%) | 1.00 | | | | | | | | | 0.85 |
| (2) Casual partner (%) | 0.30* | 1.00 | | | | | | | | 0.33 |
| (3) Heavy drinker (%) | 0.45** | -0.09 | 1.00 | | | | | | | 0.18 |
| (4) Feelings of depression (mean) | 0.12 | 0.11 | 0.50** | 1.00 | | | | | | -0.14 |
| (5) Median wages | -0.12 | 0.00 | 0.18 | 0.20 | 1.00 | | | | | -0.33 |
| (6) Recent arrival (%) | 0.34** | -0.05 | -0.23 | -0.48** | -0.27* | 1.00 | | | | 0.51 |
| (7) Non-Hispanic residents (%) | -0.26* | 0.06 | 0.17 | -0.08 | 0.43** | -0.15 | 1.00 | | | -0.38 |
| (8) Unaccompanied men (%) | 0.80** | 0.38** | 0.20 | -0.19 | -0.22 | 0.45** | -0.28* | 1.00 | | 0.89 |
| (9) Apartments with female resident (%) | -0.65** | -0.36** | -0.06 | 0.12 | 0.30* | -0.43** | 0.32** | -0.68** | 1.00 | -0.78 |

representation, reinforcing the idea that the structural context of migration, namely family separation and male over-representation, undergirds part of the association between migration and HIV risks. It is also worth noting the association between the social indicators themselves. Of the 15 correlation coefficients, over half are large and statistically significant. In particular, recent arrivals and unaccompanied men tend to live together, while neighbourhoods with women tend to have less recent arrivals, higher earners, and more non-Latinos.

Overall, the association between and among health and social disorganization indicators suggests an underlying spatial distribution that systematically concentrates risk across neighbourhoods. We next perform a common factor analysis to create a risk concentration index that can be used to identify high to low risk neighbourhoods (Table 3.2, last column). Together, the analyses highlight that risk prevalence, especially sexual risks, are not randomly distributed but rather are closely associated with the structural characteristics of Latino neighbourhoods. Among these characteristics three stand out as particularly important: the share of men who are unaccompanied, of households without female residents, and of recent arrivals.

## Mapping risk concentration

In order to assess the spatial distribution of risk across neighbourhoods, we use individual factor scores to compute a five-group typology ranging from very high to very low levels of risk concentration.[1] Table 3.3 describes the variation in

Table 3.3 Concentration of risk within Latino neighbourhoods

|  | Risk concentration level | | | | |
|  | Very high | High | Medium | Low | Very low |
| --- | --- | --- | --- | --- | --- |
| *Health and sexual risks* | | | | | |
| Use of sex worker | 39.5 (4.9) | 27.8 (8.2) | 20.8 (5.8) | 16.3 (5.2) | 7.0 (7.2) |
| Casual partner (%) | 21.9 (5.4) | 31.0 (9.1) | 24.6 (9.0) | 23.1 (8.7) | 12.3 (7.5) |
| Heavy drinker (%) | 32.5 (6.3) | 25.8 (14.7) | 24.1 (12.1) | 25.6 (11.1) | 25.5 (14.2) |
| Feelings of depression (mean) | 4.7 (0.5) | 4.9 (0.7) | 4.6 (0.5) | 4.5 (0.2) | 5.3 (0.4) |
| | | | | | |
| *Social disorganization* | | | | | |
| Median wages | 9.3 (0.8) | 9.6 (1.0) | 10.0 (0.8) | 10.1 (0.7) | 10.6 (1.5) |
| Recent arrival (%) | 54.4 (5.7) | 50.6 (14.7) | 46.7 (10.8) | 37.2 (9.3) | 34.0 (5.1) |
| Non-Hispanic residents (%) | 7.9 (10.7) | 22.0 (9.9) | 17.8 (9.0) | 33.0 (12.1) | 22.0 (15.3) |
| | | | | | |
| *Gender related migration dynamics* | | | | | |
| Unaccompanied men (%) | 79.5 (4.5) | 68.6 (3.5) | 60.0 (4.4) | 53.9 (6.9) | 36.2 (10.5) |
| Appartments with female resident (%) | 45.0 (15.8) | 52.1 (4.4) | 59.8 (9.5) | 70.2 (11.1) | 85.8 (7.2) |
| | | | | | |
| N | 5 | 7 | 10 | 6 | 4 |

health risks and social disorganization measures in our typology. Results reveal that five of our 32 neighbourhoods exhibit very high levels of risk concentration, seven are categorized as high, 10 are medium, six are low, and four have very low degree of risk concentration. While 40 per cent of men in very high-risk settings report sex worker use, the figures are only 21 and 7 per cent in medium- and very low-risk neighbourhoods, respectively. While variation in other risk behaviours is less systematic, recent arrivals are clearly concentrated in riskier neighbourhoods, as are unaccompanied men and apartments lacking women.

Figure 3.1 then maps these results, along with the per cent Latino by block with larger circles reflecting higher levels of risks. Consistent with the recent formation of the community and the decentralized mode of development in Durham, Latino neighbourhoods are generally dispersed rather than spatially contiguous, and as such do not form larger ecological areas of concentration. However, the concentration of risks across neighbourhoods follows the historical development of the Latino community in Durham. The five neighbourhoods identified as very high risk include the first Latino neighbourhoods in the area, and several cluster in East Durham. Interestingly, these neighbourhoods have long concentrated recently arrived immigrants suggesting a temporal as well as spatial continuity to risk concentration.

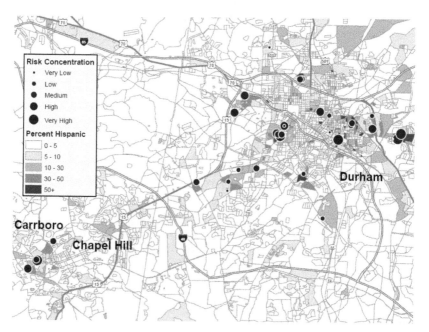

*Figure 3.1* Spatial distribution of risks across Latino neighbourhoods in Durham/Carrboro, North Carolina

### Case studies

To gain a better understanding of the mechanisms connecting neighbourhoods and health risks and how they are experienced by residents, we next draw on in-depth interviews and extensive field work in the community to illustrate three different risk environments: high (*La Maldita Vecindad*), intermediate (*Los Coloniales*), and low (The Mews).

One of the earliest areas of migrant settlement in Durham, *La Maldita Vecindad* (a neighbourhood description conferred by its residents, which translates as 'the damned/cursed neighbourhood') has been all but exclusively Latino since the mid-to late 1990s. The medium-sized complex has a reputation for both social and physical disorder. There are relatively few amenities at *La Maldita* compared with other comparably priced complexes. There is no rental office on site, so residents have to go downtown to pay their rent or put in a maintenance request, nor are there laundry, gym, or pool facilities. The only 'yard' spaces usually have cars parked on them and become very muddy when it rains. There are potholes throughout the complex as well as chipped paint, mould, and broken gutters evident along building exteriors. There is also a great deal of rubbish outside, with empty beer and soda bottles/cans strewn on the street along with copious quantities of broken glass. Apartments with broken windows are common, and residents complain of chronically poor maintenance.

In addition to this physical disorder, there is also ample evidence of social disorder in *La Maldita*, which has long served as a point of entry for newly arriving migrants. It is common for residents to take in newcomers, even if they do not know anyone in the apartment, and to provide free room and board for a couple of months while they get established. This access to immediate no-cost shelter, in addition to information on employment and ride sharing, is a critical form of social support. However, because the process concentrates recent arrivals and unaccompanied men who commonly squeeze as many as eight to 12 into a single two-bedroom apartment, it also concentrates risk. As seen in Figure 3.2 the buildings are arranged in concentric U shapes facing two common parking lots, lending it the feeling of an amphitheatre. As such, much of the social life occurs outdoors. People congregate on balconies and in parking lots, and everyone can see what everyone else is doing. Drinking alcohol outside is common; on any given evening, there are several groups of men clustered, drinking beer outside while playing cards or grilling on their balconies. It is also common for men to drink alone in public, sitting with a case of beer on one side and empty bottles on the other. Fights occasionally break out, particularly late at night, although less than before the police increased their presence there.

Public spaces in *La Maldita* are overwhelmingly the territory of men. Most men try to leave when they get more established, especially if they are able to bring their families since they feel strongly that *La Maldita* is no place for women. The few women who do live there are hardly ever seen outside – only when they leave or return to their apartments, and even then they go as quickly as possible

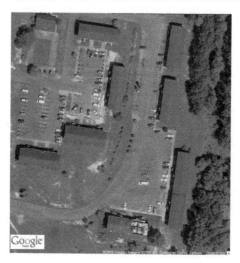

*Figure 3.2 La Maldita Vecindad*

through public areas. Women do not socialize with the men outside or at the doors of their apartments. Overall, the sense of social disorder is palpable, from the frequent presence of the purveyors of stolen goods, to loud music, to public intoxication and littering. The absence of families also contributes to an atmosphere conducive to sex worker use. It is common to see sex workers soliciting in the neighbourhood. Because of the open layout, the men readily see sex workers arrive and easily recognize them. Sex workers generally do not go door to door in *La Maldita*, but instead search out particular apartments where they had business before. They also proposition the men who are outside watching card games or socializing and even call up to men on their balconies from the parking lot below.

At *Los Coloniales*, which is characterized by an intermediate level of risk concentration, the main rental office is on site with personnel seven days a week. Maintenance requests are reported to be treated quickly. The complex also has a number of amenities, including a community service room with laundry facilities and group meeting space, a pool, and small field where residents play soccer on weekends. The town home blocks have small front and back yards that are maintained by the management. All units have marked parking spaces in front. The neighbourhood is relatively clean and well kept with a number of large trees and other landscaping, and is more racially integrated than *La Maldita*. The neighbourhood is bounded by highways and a shopping complex, and has a much more closed, less public, feeling than *La Maldita*. *Los Coloniales* was once a typical second-stage neighbourhood; a place where men moved when their wives and families joined them, to escape the rowdiness and disorder of point-of-entry neighbourhoods. Over time, as *Los Coloniales* became predominantly Latino, some of this tranquillity faded, raising the level of risk. Still, while *La Maldita* is noisy and strewn with trash, *Los Coloniales* is considerably more tranquil and cleaner. There are street vendors as in *La Maldita*, but there are no card games, hanging laundry, hawking of stolen goods, or informal street mechanics working on cars. In *Los Coloniales* people do sometimes congregate outside, but with the greater representation of families and women in the complex there is no public drinking.

Together, these elements contribute to a radically different atmosphere with respect to sex work. While sex workers are still present in *Los Coloniales*, they are far more discreet than in *La Maldita*. The location of brothels circulates among men, who generally leave the neighbourhood for commercial sex. One respondent said he preferred going to brothels because having women visit his apartment was 'embarrassing because there are many families here'. In a similar fashion, business cards claiming to be for other services but widely known to be advertising sex workers circulate, and the women who respond to the calls dress discreetly so as not to call attention to themselves and their trade. For instance, once while doing fieldwork we observed a Latina woman leaving an apartment holding a tray covered as if it had a cake. After visiting the apartment to conduct an interview, we learned that the woman was a sex worker who had come to his apartment after he called a phone number off a business card.

The Mews apartments, located in an area of more recent Latino settlement in a band of other low-risk apartment complexes in Southwest Durham offers even more contrast. Like *Los Coloniales*, the Mews apartments are very well maintained, with on-site administration and amenities such as a pool, laundry facilities, a gym, and community room. The documentation requirements to obtain an apartment are more stringent at the Mews than in *La Maldita* and even *Los Coloniales*, and the administration does not include any Spanish speakers, so it tends to attract more settled migrants with families and less unaccompanied and recently arrived men. The administration is also very active and strives to maintain order, sending written complaints to tenants who fail to abide by recycling ordinances or who leave rubbish outside. The Mews also has a full-time security guard who also lives in the neighbourhood and is strict with resident children and teenagers. While people can be seen walking their dogs and going back and forth to the administrative offices, people do not gather outside; loud music is met with rebuke, and public drinking and intoxication are not tolerated. During fieldwork here and in conversations with long-term residents, we did not uncover any sex worker presence at all in the Mews, neither distributors of business cards nor sex workers canvassing the area.

Thus, neighbourhood differences in the atmosphere of HIV risk are stark. Where recent migrants end up in Durham is generally a matter of social connections; the vast majority move in initially with a family member of friend from home. However, these connections are themselves structured by the dynamics of migration and often lead to men-only environments. For unaccompanied men newly arrived to Durham, point-of-entry communities like *La Maldita* provide critical social support, shelter, and access to employment while migrants adapt to their new environment. At the same time, however, they also concentrate disadvantage and disorder, heightening exposure to HIV risk. Migrants who arrive in *La Maldita* often find themselves isolated and depressed, cut off from family and partners, and in the midst of a male-dominated environment associated with alcohol abuse, social disorder, and permissiveness with respect to casual and commercial sex. With social networks largely comprised of other young, unaccompanied men, there are few sources of social control to discourage risk behaviours. Moreover, there are scant avenues for meeting members of the opposite sex, as few other residents of the complex are women. While most migrants living in these areas decry the poor conditions and would prefer to live somewhere else, it is not always easy to do so. Especially for the recently arrived who lack transportation and may not be able to afford rent with fewer occupants, it is often difficult to relocate. Most view their time in these communities as a sacrifice they make while saving up for their families to be able to join them, and wait for that to happen before moving to better conditions.

Migrants whose contacts lead them to less risk-concentrated settings, on the other hand, face a very different environment. Surrounded by families, women, and children, they reside in a structure of social control and support that discourages risk behaviours. Public drinking is not accepted and other types of disorder are less visible. The possibility of finding non-commercial partners is enhanced by the presence of unattached women living in the community.

## Discussion

This chapter elaborated an ecological description of HIV risk behaviour among Latino migrants that highlighted the role of neighbourhood social disorganization in concentrating social disadvantages. International migration disrupts social bonds and avenues of social control. However, there is considerable variation in the structural conditions of immigrant neighbourhoods, rendering HIV risk a collective as well as individual-level phenomenon.

Using both quantitative and qualitative information collected across 32 immigrant-receiving neighbourhoods in Durham, North Carolina our analysis documented a clear concentration of health risks in well-specified ecological areas. Behaviours such as sex worker use, multiple partnerships, and heavy drinking do not occur in isolation; instead they tend to cluster in certain neighbourhoods. This suggests that targeted health programmes to reach the rapidly growing and recently arrived Latino population could take a more holistic approach integrating different health behaviours and that policies affecting one particular aspect, such as alcohol use, could also produce spillover effects on other dimensions of well-being.

In addition, the concentration of health risks overlaps with other structural disadvantages, including low income and ethnic heterogeneity. These structural disadvantages inhibit the development of the interpersonal relationships that could protect migrants in their new environment. Moreover, the spatial pattern is not random; instead the oldest Latino neighbourhoods in Durham have the greatest concentration of recent migrants, providing continuity to the elevated health risks found there. Targeting these areas could be particularly efficacious in efforts to reduce disease transmission.

Finally, the gender composition of the migration flow acts as an added dimension of neighbourhood structural disadvantage that is directly associated with risk. While not theorized in classical social disorganization approaches, the relative under-representation of women in Latino migration translates into a context of reception that complicates partner selection for men and reduces informal channels of social control provided by women.

Results suggest that programmes and interventions need to continue to shift focus from individuals to the contexts in which they operate. The fact that health risks overlap with structural neighbourhood disadvantage, especially gender imbalances, indicates that broader processes connected with poverty and migration policies undergird much of immigrants' exposure to health risks. While politically unpopular, family reunification policies, or policies that allow families to migrate together, hold great potential for reducing HIV risk behaviour among migrant men.

In addition, results indicate that the efficacy of health interventions and programmes could be enhanced by focusing on neighbourhoods as opposed to larger community or metropolitan areas. Most community-based interventions start with an assessment of community priority health problems without clear guidelines for identifying neighbourhood processes. Targeted interventions focusing on the conditions exposing migrants to risks in particular neighbourhoods could be more efficacious and result in longer-term effects than those that fail to account for the concentration of risks in their designs.

Finally, the challenge is to be more creative in the public health policies. At the individual level there is a growing consensus that HIV interventions need to focus on men, since it is their behaviour and power within relationships that accounts for much of the diffusion of the disease. At the neighbourhood level, though, the focus should include efforts to avoid the spatial concentration of disadvantages and facilitate a more even distribution of women and families across local areas. This entails working with building managers, the police, and local advocacy organizations to mitigate the disorder that can sometimes characterize male-dominated neighbourhoods to make them more appealing to women.

## Notes

1 The cutoff points for the factor score are: very high ($> = 1$), high (0.25 to 1), medium (-0.25 to 0.25), low (-1 to -0.25), and very low ($< = -1$).

## References

Alba, R. and Nee, V. (2003) *Remaking the American Mainstream: Assimilation and Contemporary Immigration*. Cambridge: Harvard University Press.

Brody, E. B. (1970) *Behavior in New Environments: Adaptation of Migrant Populations*. Beverly Hills: Sage Publications.

Hagan, J., Simpson, J. and Gillis, A. R. (1987) 'Class in the Household: A Power-Control Theory of Gender and Delinquency', *The American Journal of Sociology*, 92:788–816.

Organista, K. C., Carrillo, H. and Ayala, G. (2004) 'HIV Prevention with Mexican Migrants: Review, Critique, and Recommendations', *Journal of Acquired Immune Deficiency Syndromes*, 37:S227–S239.

Parrado, E. A., Flippen, C. A. and McQuiston, C. (2004) 'Use of Commercial Sex Workers among Hispanic Migrants in North Carolina: Implications for the Spread of HIV', *Perspectives on Sexual and Reproductive Health*, 36(4):150–56.

Parrado, E. A., McQuiston, C. and Flippen, C. A. (2005) 'Participatory Survey Research: Integrating Community Collaboration and Quantitative Methods for the Study of Gender and HIV Risks among Hispanic Migrants', *Sociological Methods and Research*, 34:204–39.

Portes, A. and Rumbaut, R. G. (2006) *Immigrant America: A Portrait*. Berkeley: University of California Press.

Robison, J., Gruman, C., Gaztambide, S. and Blank, K. (2002) 'Screening for Depression in Middle-aged and Older Puerto Rican Primary Care Patients', *Journal of Gerontology: Medical Sciences*, 57(5):M308–14.

Sampson, R. J. (1988) 'Local Friendship Ties and Community Attachment in Mass Society: A Multilevel Systemic Model', *American Sociological Review*, 53:766–79.

Shaw, C. R. and McKay, H. D. (1942) *Juvenile Delinquency and Urban Areas*. Chicago: University of Chicago Press.

Thomas, W. I. and Znaniecki, F. (1920) *The Polish Peasant in Europe and America*. Boston: Gorham Press.

# Chapter 4

# Conflict, forced migration, sexual behaviour and HIV/AIDS

*Bayard Roberts and Preeti Patel*

Globally, there has been a significant rise in the number of conflicts over the past 50 years and this is principally due to increasing civil unrest between a country government and rebel insurgents. These conflicts are characterised by increasing disregard for humanitarian law and the deliberate targeting of civilians. The result has been the forced migration of civilian populations, either within the borders of their country as internally displaced persons (IDPs) or through crossing an internationally recognised border as refugees. Protracted conflicts over the last two decades which have resulted in large-scale forced migration, include those in Afghanistan, Angola, Burundi, Colombia, Democratic Republic of Congo, Iraq, Liberia, Mozambique, Rwanda, Sierra Leone, Somalia, Sri Lanka, Sudan, and Uganda amongst others. Forced migration is generally a long-term phenomenon with persons displaced for years and often decades. The displaced may live in camps, or be dispersed in rural or urban areas.

The number of IDPs has gradually risen while the number of refugees (both those recognised as refugees and those claiming refugee status) has fallen over the past two decades. At the beginning of the 1990s there were around 20 million IDPs and 20 million refugees. In 2007, there were around 26 million IDPs and 16 million refugees. Around 15 million of the displaced persons were in sub-Saharan Africa, and over three-quarters of these were IDPs (IDMC 2008; UNHCR 2008).

The extent to which conflict and forced migration increase vulnerability to HIV is context-specific and depends upon numerous overlapping individual, socioeconomic and epidemiological factors. These include sexual behaviour and sexual violence, gender inequality, loss of income, availability of education, living conditions, the type and the length of conflict and displacement, and access to HIV and sexual and reproductive health services. They also include the local characteristics of the HIV epidemic such as prevalence rates in areas of origin in the surrounding host community or among armed combatants, and mixing between these groups (Spiegel 2004).

The aim of this chapter is to explore how conflict and forced migration may influence vulnerability to becoming infected with HIV through altered consensual, coerced and, commercial sexual behaviour. The chapter focuses specifically on refugees and IDPs in sub-Saharan Africa given the region's high number of forcibly displaced persons and HIV prevalence. The chapter will firstly present arguments on how forced migration may increase vulnerability to HIV through altered sexual behaviour. The chapter then presents evidence on how conflict and forced migration may act as a protective factor against HIV infection. This is followed by a discussion on the research challenges and needs to help improve understanding of the complex and sometimes paradoxical effects of forced migration on sexual behaviour and HIV-related vulnerability and risk.

## Forced migration and increased vulnerability to HIV infection

Forced migration often entails breaking with family, friends, and established social networks, which in turn, can displace people from traditional norms and values and result in changing social behaviour. This can result in altered sexual behaviour, such as having consecutive and short-term sexual relationships (UNHCR/UNOCHA 2006). In a study of IDPs in Burundi, for example, displaced persons commented on the loss of social values and increasing partner change in their communities since the war and displacement (Boutin and Nkurunziza 2001).

The psychological and social effects of violence, displacement and impoverishment and the intense sense of frustration experienced may also result in risk-taking behaviour such as unprotected sex, sex with a non-regular partner or transactional sex (Khaw et al. 2000). A study of long-term Congolese refugees in Tanzania, for example, recorded higher rates of high-risk sex (sex with a non-regular partner or sex worker) among young refugees than in the surrounding population (Rowley et al. 2008). In one of the few studies on urban IDPs, Agadjanian and Avogo (2008) also reveal higher rates of high-risk sexual behaviour by IDP men than non-IDP men in Luanda, Angola.

It has been speculated that violence, displacement, poverty and the psychological *sequelae* may also lead to hazardous alcohol and drug use which could increase the likelihood of higher risk and unprotected sex (Odejide 2006; Strathdee et al. 2006). The poverty accompanying displacement can lead to forcibly displaced persons, particularly men, travelling away from their families to find work and spending times in hostels and having a greater number of sexual partners, including sex workers (Haour-Knipe et al. 1999). This may be attributable to changes in social norms compared to their home environments, a sense of isolation and loneliness, and social pressures from fellow residents including pressures to conform to masculine ideals of sexual behaviour.

Access to reproductive health and HIV prevention services and information may also be reduced by forced migration, particularly in the early emergency stages of the displacement before humanitarian agencies have mobilised a response. Lack of HIV prevention and sexual and reproductive health services can also be acute in post-conflict periods as displaced persons return. A recent

United National High Commissioner for Refugees (UNHCR) survey in Juba, Southern Sudan, for example, found that returning displaced persons and residents of Juba had low knowledge that condoms help prevent HIV and had limited access to HIV counselling and testing services (UNHCR 2007). The post-conflict period can also increase vulnerability as populations recover from the trauma of war, transport increases and voluntary migration increases in the search for work (Spiegel *et al.* 2007; Strand *et al.* 2007).

IDPs and displaced persons living outside of camps generally have less access to reproductive health and HIV services and information in comparison with camp-based refugees (IAWG 2004; UNHCR/UNOCHA 2006). This reflects the limited support and protection afforded to IDPs under international law, by the United Nations (UN), and particularly by country governments who may be responsible for the displacement itself (Goodwin-Gill 1996; UNOCHA 2004; IDMC 2008). Reforms to the humanitarian system in 2005 which sought to increase protection, support and accountability by UN agencies for IDPs may help address this, but further assistance for persons displaced outside of camps is still required from country governments and the international community (UNHCR/UNOCHA 2006; Davies 2007).

The impoverishment frequently arising from conflict and forced migration can result in forcibly displaced persons having to use sex in exchange for money and other resources (Khaw *et al.* 2000; Hankins *et al.* 2002). This may be with soldiers (active and demobilised), and peacekeepers who may carry a relatively high risk of HIV and sexually transmitted infections (Newman 2001; Patel and Tripodi 2007a). It can also be with other displaced persons.

In a study of Congolese refugees in Tanzania, for example, 92 per cent of respondents who had ever had transactional sex indicated that it occurred more often after the displacement when living in the camp than before the displacement (Rowley *et al.* 2008). Transactional sex can also take place with local populations but further investigation is required to understand the characteristics of transactional sex within displaced populations, and between displaced and host populations. Refugee and IDP children can also be vulnerable to involvement in transactional sex due to impoverishment and power imbalances with adult abusers. These power imbalances become particularly acute if the perpetrators are military, peacekeepers or aid workers (Machel 2001; Save the Children 2008).

The risk of HIV infection amongst those forced into transactional sex is influenced by factors such as the number of sexual partners and type of sexual intercourse, use of condoms, and presence of sexually transmitted infections and HIV amongst sexual partners. The level of transactional sex work may depend upon the impoverishment of the displaced population, whether displaced persons' settlements are located close to heavily populated areas, transportation routes, or other groups such as army or peacekeeping units. However, there is very little reliable evidence on the magnitude and characteristics of sex work amongst displaced persons.

Sexual violence by armed combatants is frequently reported during conflicts and displacement. Recent examples include Darfur, the Democratic Republic of Congo, Rwanda, Kosovo, Bosnia, Uganda, and Angola. Unfortunately, there are few studies that quantify the magnitude and characteristics of the sexual violence. Exceptions include a survey in Sierra Leone in which 9 per cent of 991 respondents reported one or more war-related sexual assault experiences during the war (Amowitz et al. 2002), and a survey in Liberia in which nearly half of the women and girls surveyed had been subjected to at least one act of physical or sexual violence by combatants (Swiss et al. 1998).

Factors influencing vulnerability to becoming infected with HIV through sexual violence include the severity, type and incidence of sexual attacks, the number of perpetrators, condom use, and the likelihood of sexually transmitted infections and HIV amongst the perpetrator and survivor. Some evidence suggests that armed combatants in some areas may have higher rates of HIV and sexually transmitted infections than the general civilian population (UNAIDS 1998; Newman 2001). The few studies on the behaviour of armed forces in Africa indicate that although the level of awareness about HIV among troops is relatively high, it has not made any significant impact with regards to changing high-risk sexual behaviour such as unprotected sex (Adebajo et al. 2002; van Breda 2006). Incidents of peacekeepers committing rape in the civilian populations they are mandated to protect have also been documented (Save the Children 2008). However, there is limited reliable evidence on sexual practices and prevalence of HIV and sexually transmitted infections among armed combatants and peacekeepers (Allen 2006; Barnett and Prins 2006; McInnes 2006). Nicky Dahrendrof of the UN in the Democratic Republic of Congo notes:

> anecdotal evidence [on sexual violence] is all we have and much of it is incorrect. We can't develop our peacekeeping programmes without understanding the perpetrators and victims better ... But after all these years – nothing has been done to pull the crucial data together.
>
> (cited in Bechler 2008)

Explanations of the behaviour of armed combatants who perpetrate sexual violence include using violence against women as a spoil of war, using sexual violence as a means of destroying the opponent's culture and humiliating the enemy, and also a result of pre-existing animosity towards women which is allowed to be more aggressive in the context of impunity and lawlessness (Seifert 1992). Constructions of masculinity in armies are associated with power, a sense of impunity, and a culture strongly linked with risk-taking – all of which can also increase sexual violence by armed combatants (Patel and Tripodi 2007b). High rates of sexual violence experienced by armed combatants have been recorded in Liberia and this could result in the future infliction of sexual violence by armed combatants upon civilians (Johnson et al. 2008).

Incidents of sexual violence against men and boys by armed combatants have been reported in the majority of armed conflicts during the last decade (Russell 2007). Explanations for sexual violence against males include issues of power, dominance, and emasculation (Sivakumaran 2007). However, there are few studies which present data on the rates of sexual violence experienced by men and boys and little is known about the scope or nature of sexual violence by men against other men or about the psychosocial consequences for survivors (Russell 2007).

Reports also suggest sexual violence by intimate partners and known persons may be more common than sexual violence from armed combatants in long-term situations of displacement where the risk of attacks by armed combatants is reduced (McGinn 2000; Rowley *et al.* 2008). A study in Southern Sudan, for example, noted how war-related psycho-social problems, unemployment and loss of livelihoods, frustration, and a sense of emasculation amongst displaced men fostered behavioural changes and sexual violence (ISIS-WICCE 2007). The sexual violence may also be fuelled by increasing alcohol or substance abuse. Studies of displaced populations in Uganda, for example, have noted increased alcohol use contributing to domestic sexual violence (El-Bushra 2000; Baron 2002). However, further research is required on the magnitude and characteristics of sexual violence by intimate partners and known persons amongst displaced persons.

Arguments that sexual violence during conflict and displacement increase HIV prevalence at the population level have also been rejected on the basis that they use unreliable data and that even widespread rape is unlikely to result in a population-level change in HIV prevalence. However, this should not be interpreted to say that widespread rape does not pose serious risks to women's acquisition of HIV on an individual basis or in specific settings (Anema *et al.* 2008).

## Evidence of forced migration as a protective factor against HIV infection

Despite the numerous factors arising from forced migration that may increase vulnerability to becoming infected with HIV, evidence also suggests that in some circumstances, conflict may actually act as a protective factor against HIV transmission (Strand *et al.* 2007). HIV prevalence rates among forcibly displaced persons in many areas of sub-Saharan Africa are generally lower than the surrounding populations, and there is no evidence that they exacerbate the HIV epidemic in surrounding communities (Spiegel *et al.* 2007). A general explanation is that displaced persons often come from rural areas which tend to have lower HIV rates than more heavily populated areas (*ibid*).

There are a number of factors related to sexual behaviour that may help to explain these findings. Displaced persons living in camps are often limited in their movements because of insecurity, restrictions by camp authorities, and impoverishment (Fabiani *et al.* 2007). This disrupts traditional social networks, particularly along transport routes which are often catalysts in the spread of HIV and may in turn result in lower exposure to HIV (Spiegel *et al.* 2007; Strand *et al.*

2007). It is also suggested that the psychological consequences of conflict and forced migration may reduce sexual desire and activity (Mock *et al.* 2004; Mulanga *et al.* 2004), although this requires further investigation.

Displaced persons may also have lower purchasing power than prior to the conflict and compared to surrounding communities which may reduce their interactions with sex workers (Mock *et al.* 2004; Mulanga *et al.* 2004). As noted above, however, this impoverishment may increase the likelihood of some displaced persons themselves turning to commercial sex for income.

Some displaced persons, particularly refugees living in camps, have greater access to reproductive health and HIV/AIDS services and information than before they arrived in the camps and also compared to surrounding communities (Spiegel 2004). The results of HIV behavioural surveys conducted by UNHCR generally show higher exposure to HIV information programmes, and utilisation of counselling and testing facilities than in surrounding communities (UNHCR/GLIA 2004, 2006; Rowley *et al.* 2008).

## Research challenges and needs

Better understanding of how forced migration may alter sexual behaviour and vulnerability to HIV is impeded by the lack of reliable and rigorous research on the subject, particularly for IDPs and displaced persons not living in camps. The resultant impact can be ineffective programming and misinformed reports which risk stigmatising displaced persons as vectors of disease (Lowicki-Zucca *et al.* 2005; Allen 2006).

The limited amount of reliable data on forcibly displaced persons is due in part to the substantial challenges associated with conducting research in conflict-affected areas which may be characterised by insecurity, political constraints, restricted access to populations, public fear and mistrust, and a lack of infra-structure, money and other resources. Displaced persons not living in camps may also be difficult to locate and identify, and may be reluctant to participate in research. In addition, national governments are often reluctant to address the needs of forced migrant populations and so may not be able or willing to pro-vide information or support, particularly for IDPs who may be opposed by the government. Even in Uganda, which for a period was viewed as a model of best practice in HIV prevention, limited data existed for its large forcibly displaced populations (Salama and Dondero 2001; Allen 2006). The post-conflict period when displaced persons return to their home areas can also be characterised by weak health systems that are unable to support reliable research on HIV and AIDS (Johnson *et al.* 2005). The very weak data on sexual behaviour and HIV pre-valence in the military is partly attributable to the fact that it is considered sen-sitive for national security reasons and therefore is not readily accessible. Access to rebel armies and groups such as demobilised soldiers is particularly difficult.

The sensitivity and stigma frequently associated with researching sexual behaviour, particularly in relation to HIV, pose significant methodological challenges (Cleland *et al.* 2004; Plummer *et al.* 2004). Survivors of sexual violence may also feel a sense of shame, humiliation, fear of retaliation, and reluctance to discuss such painful events (Ellsberg and Heise 2005; Mills *et al.* 2006). These challenges may result in refusal to participate in research or misreporting of sexual behaviour resulting in biased results. These challenges can be additionally complex when researching the sexual violence experienced by men. In many settings, dominant understandings of masculinity are often incompatible with the victimization of men, and so research is not instigated (Del Zotto and Jones 2002). This may be further compounded by humanitarian workers and researchers internalising stereotypical gender roles with men as perpetrators of violence and women as victims (Donnelly 1996; Carpenter 2006). In addition, sexual activity between men is taboo in many societies and therefore reports of same-sex sexual violence can be extremely low (Oosterhoff *et al.* 2004).

Subjects as sensitive and intimate as sexual behaviour and relations are not easily researched. Rigorous in-depth studies may be required for studying individual situations of forced migration. They provide an essential way of strengthening knowledge of local conceptions and attitudes towards sexual behaviour and decision-making amongst displaced persons and related populations such as soldiers and peacekeepers, particularly on taboo subjects such as rape and anal sex. Such methods could help explore how social, cultural and moral norms, including gender and power relations, are influenced by forced migration and what effect this has upon sexual behaviour.

Lessons can be learned from stable settings where studies on sexuality show how cultural conceptions of sexuality, gender and trust have an important effect on their actions (Hansjorg 2003). Knowledge on HIV-related stigma and discrimination experienced by displaced persons is also extremely weak. Work on conceptualising stigma and exploring its origins, development and responses (Parker and Aggleton 2003) could be applied in situations of forced migration. Interdisciplinary studies can also make an important contribution, and comparative analysis of studies using different research methods could help to validate findings and interpret data with greater understanding and insight.

Systematically recorded HIV behavioural surveillance data of displaced populations and surrounding communities are required. However, such quantitative data are currently limited, particularly for IDPs and non-camp populations. They can also be methodologically flawed, weakened by small sample sizes and limited precision, lack of field-testing, and poor translation processes (Spiegel and Le 2006). Initiatives to systematise the methods and standards for HIV behavioural surveys are to be welcomed (UNHCR/GLIA/World Bank 2008). Such work would also support the use of comparative and meta-analyses studies.

Longitudinal quantitative studies are required to show the influence of conflict and migration on sexual behaviour and HIV incidence, including comparisons with surrounding populations, and also in post-conflict periods given the concerns over increased vulnerability in post-conflict situations (Spiegel *et al.* 2007; Strand *et al.* 2007). Such studies are methodologically complex and require political and financial support but may nevertheless be possible in certain contexts. Comparative quantitative studies on sexual behaviour amongst forced migrants and surrounding populations may also be valuable in strengthening understanding of how migration affects sexual behaviour and HIV vulnerability (Agadjanian and Avogo 2008; Rowley *et al.* 2008).

Finally, there remains a critical need to improve understanding of the impact and effectiveness of HIV-related programmes and interventions. Few studies have systematically looked at the impact and effectiveness of interventions for sexual behaviour in conflict and post-conflict situations. The challenges of assessing impact of interventions addressing sexual behaviour, and sexual violence in particular, are clearly difficult given the extremely sensitive nature of the subject matter and the complex and fluid nature of many refugees' and IDPs' environments. However, assessment guidelines do exist (WHO/UNFPA/UNHCR 1999; Marsh 2005). The methodological experiences and ethical considerations from research in more stable settings on sexual behaviour and sexual violence could also be harnessed for work with forcibly displaced populations (Cleland *et al.* 2004; Plummer *et al.* 2004; Ellsberg and Heise 2005).

## Conclusions

This chapter has described the numerous factors arising from forced migration which may influence sexual behaviour and vulnerability to HIV infection. These factors vary in significance depending on the local situation and context. However, evidence indicates that in general, HIV prevalence does not necessarily increase in areas affected by conflict and that forcibly displaced persons are not at heightened risk of transmitting HIV. The chapter also noted a series of research limitations and needs on the subject of forced migration, sexual behaviour and HIV vulnerability. There are clear dangers arising from the scarcity of reliable evidence which can result in ill-informed decision-making and ineffective HIV programming for displaced and surrounding populations. The scarcity of evidence can also feed myths which may further stigmatise displaced populations and increase discrimination against them.

## References

Adebajo, S., Mafeni, J., Moreland, S. and Murray, N. (2002) *Knowledge, Attitudes, and Sexual Behaviour among the Nigerian Military Concerning HIV/AIDS and STDS*, Lagos: Armed Forces Programme on AIDS Control/USAID.

Agadjanian, V. and Avogo, W. (2008) 'Forced migration and HIV/AIDS', *International Migration*, 46(3): 189–216.

Allen, T. (2006) 'AIDS and evidence: interrogating some Ugandan myths', *Journal of Biosocial Science*, 38(1): 7–28.

Amowitz, L., Reis, C. Lyons, H., Vann, B., Mansaray, B., Akinsulure-Smith, A., Taylor, L. and Iacopino, V. (2002) 'Prevalence of war-related sexual violence and other human rights abuses among internally displaced persons in Sierra Leone', *Journal of the American Medical Association*, 287(4): 513–21.

Anema, A., Joffres, M. R., Mills, E. and Spiegel, P. B. (2008) 'Widespread rape does not directly appear to increase the overall HIV prevalence in conflict-affected countries: so now what?' *Emerging Themes in Epidemiology*, 5: 11.

Barnett, T. and Prins, G. (2006) 'HIV/AIDS and security: fact, fiction and evidence', *International Affairs*, 82(2): 359–68.

Baron, N. (2002) 'Community based psychosocial and mental health services for Southern Sudanese refugees in long term exile in Uganda', J. De Jong (ed.) *Trauma, War, and Violence: Public Mental Health in Socio-Cultural Context*, New York: Kluwer Academic/ Plenum Publishers.

Bechler, R. (2008) 'Sexual violence: not just a gender issue'. Online. Available from: www.opendemocracy.net/blog/rosemary-bechler/2008/06/05/sexual-violence-not-just-a-gender-issue (accessed 4 December 2008).

Boutin, G. and Nkurunziza, S. (2001) 'Burundi: developing strategies for self-reliance. A study of displacement in four provinces', M. Vincent and B. Sorensen (eds) *Caught Between Borders: Response Strategies of the Internally Displaced*, London: Pluto Press.

Carpenter, R. (2006) 'Recognising gender-based violence against civilian men and boys in conflict situations', *Security Dialogue*, 37(1): 83–103.

Cleland, J., Boerma, J. T., Carael, M. and Weir, S. S. (2004) 'Monitoring sexual behaviour in general populations: a synthesis of lessons of the past decade', *Sexually Transmitted Infections*, 80(Suppl 2): ii1–7.

Davies, A. (2007) 'Is humanitarian reform improving IDP protection and assistance?', *Forced Migration Review*, 29: 15–16.

Del Zotto, A. and Jones, A. 'Male-on-male sexual violence in wartime: human rights' last taboo?', Paper presented at the annual convention of the International Studies Association, New Orleans, 23–27 March 2002.

Donnelly, D. K. S. (1996) '"Honey, we don't do men": gender stereotypes and the provision of services to sexually assaulted males', *Journal of Interpersonal Violence*, 11: 441–48.

El-Bushra, J. (2000) *Transforming Conflict: Some Thoughts on a Gendered Understanding of Conflict Processes*, London: Zed Press.

Ellsberg, M. and Heise, L. (2005) *Researching Violence Against Women: A Practical Guide for Researchers and Activists*, Geneva: World Health Organisation/Path.

Fabiani, M., Nattabi, B., Pierotti, C., Ciantia, F., Opio, A. A., Musinguzi, J., Ayella, E. O. and Declich, S. (2007) 'HIV-1 prevalence and factors associated with infection in the conflict-affected region of North Uganda', *Conflict and Health*, 1: 3.

Goodwin-Gill, G. (1996) *The Refugee in International Law*, Oxford: Clarendon Press.

Hankins, C. A., Friedman, S. R. Zafar, T. and Strathdee, S. A. (2002) 'Transmission and prevention of HIV and sexually transmitted infections in war settings: implications for current and future armed conflicts', *AIDS*, 16(17): 2245–52.

Hansjorg, D. (2003) 'Sexuality, AIDS, and the lures of modernity: reflexivity and morality among young people in rural Tanzania', *Medical Anthropology*, 22: 23–52.

Haour-Knipe, M., Leshabari, M. and Lwihula, G. (1999) 'Interventions for workers away from their families', L. Gibney, R. J. DiClemente, S. H. Vermund (eds) *Preventing HIV in Developing Countries: Biomedical and Behavioral Approaches*, New York: Kluwer Academic/ Plenum Press.

IAWG (2004) *Inter-Agency Global Evaluation of Reproductive Health Services for Refugees and Internally Displaced Persons*, Geneva: Inter Agency Working Group.

IDMC (2008) *Internal Displacement: Global Overview of Trends and Developments in 2007*, Geneva: Internal Development Monitoring Centre.

ISIS-WICCE (2007) *Women's Experiences During Armed Conflict in Southern Sudan, 1983–2005: The Case of Juba County Central Equatorial State*, Kampala: Isis-WICCE 2007.

Johnson, K., Asher, J., Rosborough, S., Raja, A., Panjabi, R., Beadling, C. and Lawry, L. (2008) 'Association of combatant status and sexual violence with health and mental health outcomes in post-conflict Liberia', *Journal of the American Medical Association*, 300 (6): 676–90.

Johnson, K., Kennedy, S. B., Harris, A. O., Lincoln, A., Neace, W. and Collins, D. (2005) 'Strengthening the HIV/AIDS service delivery system in Liberia: an international research capacity-building strategy', *Journal of Evaluation in Clinical Practice*, 11(3): 257–73.

Khaw, A. J., Salama, P., Burkholder, B. and Dondero, T. J. (2000) 'HIV risk and prevention in emergency-affected populations: a review', *Disasters*, 24(3): 181–97.

Lowicki-Zucca, M., Spiegel, P. and Ciantia, F. (2005) 'AIDS, conflict and the media in Africa: risks in reporting bad data badly', *Emerging Themes in Epidemiology*, 2: 12.

Machel, G. (2001) *The Impact of Armed Conflict on Children: A Critical Review of Progress Made and Obstacles Encountered in Increasing Protection for War-Affected Children, 1996–2000*, New York: UNICEF.

Marsh, M. (2005) *Methods and Systems for the Assessment and Monitoring of Sexual Violence and Exploitation in Conflict Situations*, New York: Social Science Research Council, UNFPA, WHO.

McGinn, T. (2000) 'Reproductive health of war-affected populations: what do we know?', *International Family Planning Perspectives*, 26(4): 174–80.

McInnes, C. (2006) 'HIV/AIDS and security', *International Affairs*, 82(2): 315–26.

Mills, E. J., Singh, S., Nelson, B. D. and Nachega, J. B. (2006) 'The impact of conflict on HIV/AIDS in sub-Saharan Africa', *International Journal of STD & AIDS*, 17(11): 713–17.

Mock, N. B., Duale, S., Brown, L. F., Mathys, E., O'Maonaigh, H. C., Abul-Husn, N. K. and Elliott, S. (2004) 'Conflict and HIV: A framework for risk assessment to prevent HIV in conflict-affected settings in Africa', *Emerging Themes in Epidemiology*, 1(1): 6.

Mulanga, C., Bazepeo, S. E., Mwamba, J. K., Butel, C., Tshimpaka, J. W., Kashi, M., Lepira, F., Caraël, M., Peeters, M. and Delaporte, E. (2004) 'Political and socioeconomic instability: how does it affect HIV? A case study in the Democratic Republic of Congo', *AIDS*, 18(5): 832–34.

Newman, L. M. (2001) 'HIV seroprevalence among military blood donors in Manica Province, Mozambique', *International Journal of STD & AIDS*, 12(4): 278–79.

Odejide, A. O. (2006) 'Status of Drug Use/Abuse in Africa: A Review', *International Journal of Mental Health and Addiction*, 4(2): 87–102.

Oosterhoff, P., Zwanikken, P. and Ketting, E. (2004) 'Sexual torture of men in Croatia and other conflict situations: an open secret', *Reproductive Health Matters*, 12(23): 68–77.

Parker, R. and Aggleton, P. (2003) 'HIV and AIDS-related stigma and discrimination: a conceptual framework and implications for action', *Social Science & Medicine*, 57(1): 13–24.

Patel, P. and Tripodi, P. (2007a) 'Peacekeepers, HIV and the role of masculinity in military behaviour', *International Peacekeeping*, 14(5): 584–98.

Patel, P. and Tripodi, P. (2007b) 'Linking HIV to Peacekeepers', R. Ostergard (ed.) *HIV/AIDS and the Threat to National and International Security*, Basingstoke: Palgrave Macmillan.

Plummer, M. L., Ross, D. A., Wight, D., Changalucha, J., Mshana, G., Wamoyi, J., Todd, J., Anemona, A., Mosha, F. F., Obasi, A. I. and Hayes, R. J. (2004) '"A bit more truthful": the validity of adolescent sexual behaviour data collected in rural northern Tanzania using five methods', *Sexually Transmitted Infections*, 80(Suppl 2): ii49–56.

Rowley, E., Spiegel, P., Tunze, Z., Mbaruku, G., Schilperoord, M. and Njogu, P. (2008) 'Differences in HIV-related behaviors at Lugufu refugee camp and surrounding host villages, Tanzania', *Conflict and Health* 2(13). Available from: www.pubmedcentral.nih. gov/picrender.fcgi?artid=2596783&blobtype=pdf (accessed 29 May 2009).

Russell, W. (2007) 'Sexual violence against men and boys', *Forced Migration Review*, 27:22–23.

Salama, P. and Dondero, T. J. (2001) 'HIV surveillance in complex emergencies', *AIDS*, 15(Suppl 3): S4–12.

Save the Children (May 2008) *No One to Turn to: The Under-Reporting of Child Sexual Exploitation and Abuse by Aid Workers and Peacekeepers*, London: Save the Children.

Seifert, R. (1992) *War and Rape. Analytical Approaches*, Geneva: Women's International League for Peace and Freedom.

Sivakumaran, S. (2007) 'Sexual violence against men in armed conflict', *European Journal of International Law*, 18(2): 253–76.

Spiegel, P. B. (2004) 'HIV/AIDS among conflict-affected and displaced populations: dispelling myths and taking action', *Disasters*, 28(3): 322–39.

Spiegel, P. B., Bennedsen, A. R., Claass, J., Bruns, L., Patterson, N., Yiweza, D. and Schilperoord, M. (2007) 'Prevalence of HIV infection in conflict-affected and displaced people in seven sub-Saharan African countries: a systematic review', *Lancet*, 369(9580): 2187–95.

Spiegel, P. B. and Le, P. V. (2006) 'HIV behavioural surveillance surveys in conflict and post-conflict situations: A call for improvement', *Global Public Health*, 1(2): 147–156.

Strand, R. T., Fernandes Dias, L., Bergstrom, S. and Andersson, S. (2007) 'Unexpected low prevalence of HIV among fertile women in Luanda, Angola: does war prevent the spread of HIV?' *International Journal of STD & AIDS*, 18(7): 467–71.

Strathdee, S. A., Stachowiak, J. A., Todd, C. S., Al-Delaimy, W. K., Wiebel, W., Hankins, C. and Patterson, T. L. (2006) 'Complex emergencies, HIV, and substance use: no "big easy" solution', *Substance Use & Misuse*, 41(10–12): 1637–51.

Swiss, S., Jennings, P. J., Aryee, G. V., Brown, G. H., Jappah-Samukai, R. M., Kamara, M. S., Schaack, R. D. and Turay-Kanneh, R. S. (1998) 'Violence against women during the Liberian civil conflict', *Journal of the American Medical Association*, 279(8): 625–29.

UNAIDS (1998) *AIDS and the Military. UNAIDS Point of View. Best Practice Collection*, Geneva: UNAIDS.

UNHCR (2007) *HIV Behavioural Surveillance Survey Juba Municipality, South Sudan*, Geneva: UNHCR, Great Lakes Initiative, World Bank.

—— (2008) *2007 Global Trends: Refugees, Asylum-seekers, Returnees, Internally Displaced and Stateless Persons*, Geneva: UNHCR.

UNHCR/GLIA (2004) *Behavioural Surveillance Surveys among Refugees and Surrounding Host Population, Kakuma, Kenya*. Nairobi: UNHCR/GLIA.

——(2006) *HIV and AIDS Behavioural Surveillance Survey: Refugee Camps and Hosting Communities in Kawambwa and Mporokoso, Zambia*, Nairobi: UNHCR/GLIA.

UNHCR/GLIA/World Bank (2008) *Manual for Conducting HIV Behavioral Surveillance Surveys among Displaced Populations and their Surrounding Communities*, Geneva: UNHCR, Great Lakes Initiative, World Bank.

UNHCR/UNOCHA (2006) *HIV/AIDS and Internally Displaced Persons in Eight Priority Countries*, Geneva: Office of the United Nations High Commissioner for Refugees and Office for the Coordination of Humanitarian Affairs.

UNOCHA (2004) *OCHA External Evaluation of the Internal Displacement Unit*, Geneva: OCHA.

van Breda, A. (2006) 'What do our members know about HIV and AIDS?', *SA Soldier* November: 34–35.

WHO/UNFPA/UNHCR (1999) *Reproductive Health in Refugee Situations*, Geneva: WHO/UNFPA/UNHCR.

# Chapter 5

# Negotiating migration, gender and sexuality

## Health and social services for HIV-positive people from minority ethnic backgrounds in Sydney

*Henrike Körner*

If advances in biomedicine have transformed HIV infection into a chronic condition, managing a chronic condition requires access to health care and social services. Such access is directly determined by a patient's legal status as a citizen or resident of a country, and is also inextricably linked to ethnicity, language, gender and sexual orientation. In addition, studies from several countries have shown that health services for people with HIV also have an important social function, providing emotional support (Jorgensen and Marwit 2001; Anderson and Doyal 2004) and sometimes even becoming substitute family (Shedlin and Shulman 2004). Migrant women, in particular, may rely heavily on health and social services for physical, social and emotional support (Chin and Kroesen 1999; Doyal and Anderson 2006).

Sexual orientation and language affect access to health and social services in complex ways. As just one example, Caucasian gay men in the USA tend to be self-directed in their use of such services, exercising a high degree of control and actively involved with service organizations. For Spanish-speaking women, in contrast, the perception of HIV as socially unacceptable can make it extremely awkward for them to approach HIV services directly: their access was driven by agencies (Takahashi and Rodriguez 2002). In Australia, gay men tend to use gay-identified doctors, and HIV-positive gay men prefer physicians with a high HIV case load (Fogarty *et al.* 2003, 2006) whereas HIV-positive heterosexuals mainly use sexual health clinics and hospitals, and have little or no contact with other HIV services (Persson *et al.* 2006). Asian gay men in Australia make less use of sexual health services than do their Anglo-Australian counterparts (Mao *et al.* 2003). Other data from Australia suggest that migrants from non-English-speaking countries have less contact with health services before they are diagnosed with HIV: they are more likely than Australians to be diagnosed for HIV late (McDonald *et al.* 2003) and are more likely to develop AIDS (Dore *et al.* 2001).

This paper uses data from in-depth interviews with 28 HIV-positive men and women living in Australia but born in Asia, South America and southern Europe, to explore how they negotiate migration status, language, gender and sexual orientation in their quest for the health and social services.

## Theoretical framework

Individualism/collectivism (Triandis *et al.* 1988; Triandis 1995) and the notions of the independent and the interdependent self (Markus and Kitayama 1991, 1994; Kitayama *et al.* 1997) serve as the theoretical framework for this study. In individualist societies, the self is construed as autonomous, independent and separate from others. Behaviour is organized around one's own feelings, thoughts and actions. In collectivist cultures, on the other hand, the self is construed as fundamentally interdependent, as self-in-relation-to-others. An individual's thoughts, feelings and actions are contingent on the thoughts, feelings and actions of others. The interdependent self is perceived as creating and expecting mutuality. Both types of culture have notions of self-reliance and interdependence, but their meanings differ fundamentally. In individualist cultures, self-reliance means doing one's own thing and competing with others. In collectivist cultures, self-reliance means not being a burden on the in-group, usually the family. Inter-dependence in individualist cultures is understood as a utilitarian form of social exchange, whereas in collectivist cultures interdependence entails duties and obligations. Although the individualist and collectivist characteristics of cultures may coexist to various degrees and may also change, very broadly speaking Anglo-Celtic, northern and western European cultures can be characterized as predominantly individualist, whereas many Latin American, Asian, African and southern European cultures can be characterized as predominantly collectivist.

Individualism/collectivism and notions of the independent/interdependent self affect interactions with health systems. Patient-centred medicine in resource-rich Western countries focuses on the individual, on autonomy and choice, and on giving patients opportunities to be actively involved in decisions about their treatment (Mead and Bower 2000), especially when managing chronic disease (Holman and Lorig 2000). In HIV medicine, in particular, gay activists have demanded to be actively involved in decisions about their health (Epstein 1995). This model of the doctor–patient relationship cannot be applied across cultures, however (Ishikawa and Yamazaki 2005), as cultural norms concerning family responsibility, privacy, and the self-in-relation-to-others may work against the individual making choices without considering the kinship group (Leong and Lau 2001). For migrants, in addition, lack of fluency in the language of the destination country, and limited control over their material circumstances, may also constrain their ability to make decisions (Anderson *et al.* 1995). Migrants from resource-poor countries, finally, may never have encountered the concept of 'choice' in health care since they have had no resources to choose from, or not enough resources.

## Methods and study participants

Participants for the study were recruited among clients of the Multicultural HIV/AIDS and Hepatitis C Service (MHAHS) and a sexual health clinic in

Sydney, Australia. MHAHS provides clinical support to people from culturally and linguistically diverse backgrounds through bilingual/bicultural workers (called 'co-workers') from more than 20 language backgrounds. The sexual health clinic has a high HIV caseload and holds special consultations in several Asian languages. Criteria for inclusion in the study were having been born in a non-English-speaking country or speaking a language other than English at home. Respondents came from cultures that can be characterized as predominantly collectivist, and had migrated to a predominantly individualist culture. They lived in Sydney, a city with many ethnic communities – some large and some small – with formal and informal structures and networks, and also a large gay community.

This chapter uses data from interviews with 28 migrants, aged 29 to 58, including seven women, 15 gay-identified men, and six heterosexual men. They were born in 16 countries in Asia, South America and Southern Europe, and arrived in Australia between 1973 and 2001. Their reasons for and circumstances of migration have been discussed elsewhere (Körner 2007b). Three gay men had received their HIV diagnosis in their country of birth, whereas the others were diagnosed in Australia between 1984 and 2003 (Körner 2007a). At the time of the study, 11 participants were permanent residents or Australian citizens. Five had uncertain migration status when they were diagnosed, but were later granted permanent residency. The migration status of the remainder of the study participants was uncertain or precarious.

## Health services

Australia has a vast array of visas entailing different entitlements to work, as well as to health and social services. The country's national health system provides free or subsidized health care, and subsidized medication, for Australian citizens and permanent residents, as well as for people with certain visas and for asylum seekers meeting certain criteria. All of the study participants had access to clinics, to general practitioners and other health professionals, and to HIV treatment at the time of the study. They usually acted in accordance with the individualist orientation in their use of health services, that is, they sought the best outcome for themselves. Making decisions about health as an independent, autonomous individual was difficult for new migrants, however, since they were unfamiliar with the health services. Some were not quite sure to what services they had been referred. Lack of fluency in English may have contributed to their confusion, but so did the system of referral to specialized health services, and the notion of 'choice' in using health care services.

> I get mixed up myself about this centre. … I come here to get medicine. … I don't know exactly the name [of the service] … [I go there] to see the doctor and get the prescription and get the medicine from the pharmacy and blood tests.
>
> (Boupha, Cambodian woman, aged 40)[1]

HIV-positive people in Western countries often want to be actively involved in decisions about their treatment, and health professionals expect them to be so (Marelich *et al.* 2002), but participants in this study were not familiar with this kind of clinical interaction. For new migrants, problems with English and with medical jargon, and also the lack of social networks added to their difficulties in enacting the independent autonomous self.

> I had to [go on treatment] because ... because I don't have anyone ... I have to do everything by myself. ... I didn't have anyone [else] to ask any question or get any information, and then only was the doctor, and I had to go with doctor. I didn't have any choice, you know.
>
> (Habib, Cypriot gay man, aged 40)

There were also differences across gender and sexual orientation. Women's use of health services was driven mainly by others, typically by referrals from, and at the initiative of, health and social workers. For example, one Cambodian woman, diagnosed when she applied for permanent residency in Australia, and who as yet spoke no English, and did not know the difference between HIV and AIDS, said:

> And they ask me 'Did you want to come to [sexual health] clinic. There's a new place.' Then they refer me to [sexual health] clinic and there is a friend that I know. They took me to [sexual health] clinic.
>
> (Champei, Cambodian woman, aged 33)

Making choices about treatment requires sufficient information about the options available, and means discussing these options with a health care professional, a task that is difficult or impossible for migrants who have neither the necessary knowledge nor sufficient English. Here, gay men relied less on others, and showed more individualist self-reliance in finding their way around the service landscape in spite of language difficulties.

> For me the only thing is the [language] barrier because everybody here, all the person, they normally everybody friendly. ... They give all information you need ... but if you can't speak English, what they can do? Feel block again. What can you do? 'Have to hang around and talk with who?' 'You must to call here ... and call here [when you are referred to different services].' ... It's too complex, too complex.
>
> (Ricardo, Colombian gay man, aged 45)

While medical care was considered important and highly appreciated by all participants, women were concerned about confidentiality and limited their use of health services to those that were absolutely essential. Some women did not use the services of the health care interpreters available to facilitate communication with health professionals: they were afraid that the interpreters would gossip and disclose their HIV status, thus jeopardizing their inter-dependence with their communities. Concerns about confidentiality and inter-dependence with their ethnic communities also made some women travel long distances to clinics where they were less likely to encounter people they knew. The following explanation was encountered in one clinic.

> [Co-worker (translating)] She doesn't really want to go [to a regional clinic in another town] because there's a lot of Macedonian people work in the hospitals ... [even if] she doesn't live here anymore she still prefers to come [here to Sydney].
>
> (Sofija, Macedonian woman, aged 44)

A collectivist cultural orientation was also evident in women's use of mental health services. In collectivist cultures, disclosure of personal information outside the kinship group is perceived to bring shame on the family, thus making it quite problematic to open up to a counsellor (Leong and Lau 2001).

> I saw counsellor first time after [I] knew that [I] got this condition. ... Talking to someone is alright. Temporary company. But I think I have to look after myself.
>
> (Amporn, Thai woman, aged 31)

## Social services

Australian national and state governments provide access to public housing for people with low incomes, and social security payments to those with disabilities and unable to work. These benefits are available to Australian citizens and per-manent residents, and to some refugees and holders of humanitarian visas. There is a two-year waiting period for new migrants. Study participants' use of social services was, in the first instance, contingent on their migration status and entitlement. Participants entitled to public housing, social security payments, and other benefits, were very appreciative of the support they received. Meeting basic survival needs was a prerequisite for learning to live with HIV, and getting a sense for the future.

> I think that I am a very lucky person. Like this government got a very good programme for HIV people because I got good support and is very impor-tant, life style, because if you have to worry about where are you going to sleep. I think this is one of the most important things, you have a place to live. And I am doing my course – doing full-time study. I got [financial help for full-time students]. That, you know, is something too.
>
> (Roberto, Colombian gay man, aged 37)

Gay men, heterosexual men and women positioned themselves differently in their use of the services to which they were entitled. Women were more motivated by the collectivist notion of interdependence and self-reliance, guided by their duties as wives and mothers and their obligations to their families. Just as they had with health services, women limited their use of social services in order to avoid disclosure of their HIV status.

> [Co-worker (translating)] She said like, she doesn't want to go to too many services ... probably because she's Macedonian ... like she doesn't want people to know her, that she's infected. ... She doesn't really like coming to this area that much because at the time when her husband was sick and died [from AIDS-related illness] the whole community knew about it.
>
> (Sofija, Macedonian woman, aged 44)

Heterosexual men drew on both individualist and collectivist notions of interdependence. Those with young children organized their use of social services around the collectivist orientation of interdependence: they wanted to protect their children and to maintain harmony between family and ethnic community. In addition, since participants could not necessarily count on support from their extended families, they specifically wanted help to ensure their children's future. In social contexts that did not involve the family; however, some heterosexual men positioned themselves according to the individualist orientation of interdependence. Not using social services allowed them to feel free to act as they pleased, to organize their behaviours around their own wishes and desires.

> [Co-worker (translating)] It affect him a bit, but he try not to take it serious. ... [He] try to lead a normal life. Not to restrict his lifestyle. ... He have seen people who once they found out they had HIV become serious and depressed. Then that person always get worse. So, that's what he's learned from other people with HIV.
>
> (Ananda, Thai heterosexual man, aged 32)

Gay men appeared to have the greatest degree of cultural flexibility in the way they used social services, drawing on the independent and the interdependent selves in different contexts. On the one hand, some gay men limited their use of social services to the minimum in order to avoid disclosure and to protect the family's reputation. At the same time, they took advantage of the individualist orientation of Anglo-Australian society, where they could be free to act according to their own wishes. This meant that they also acted in line with the individualist orientation of self-reliance. The individualist and collectivist orientations complemented each other for gay men: independence and the individualist orientation to self-reliance enabled them to maintain a collectivist interdependent relationship with their families.

SOM: I feel more comfortable to live here in Australia rather than Thailand … Because I know that Western culture they not care much about personal matter. They don't have a gossip culture like Thailand. … And no one care about your personal life and they respect you more. …

INTERVIEWER: There are also people who would argue that this anonymity makes life more difficult in the Western world because we're not so connected. …

SOM: Yes, that's why I have to be self-reliant on myself. Happiness from myself. That's why I practise yoga and meditation because I don't depend my happiness on others. I am very happy working by myself, you know, self-reliant happiness rather than 'Oh I have to talk with people for happiness'.

(Som, Thai gay man, aged 33)

## HIV community organizations

Heterosexual participants' contact with HIV community organizations was minimal. They were often unfamiliar with such organizations, even if they had lived in Australia for a long time: some had never heard of them, and others got services and organizations mixed up. While a few used HIV organizations for assistance with financial and practical matters, they did not use the related support groups. Some were not familiar with the concept of a 'support group', and others did not feel comfortable talking about personal issues with strangers.

Gay men once again had the greatest flexibility in their cultural positioning: independence and interdependence according to cultural background, or interdependence according to sexual orientation. Interdependence with gay community and HIV groups was problematic for some, however. Some participated in gay community groups, but others who had attended HIV-positive support groups – especially Asian gay men – experienced exclusion and discontinued their involvement.

SUNAN: I went to the [group] … but I feel that they are not for Asian type people. … I don't feel comfortable at all.

INTERVIEWER: Can you try and describe why you don't feel comfortable there?

SUNAN: I think they talk to each other. Australian they talk to each other. … So I feel isolated.

(Sunan, Thai gay man, aged 33)

For some gay men interdependence with gay HIV-positive groups did not work because there was too much talk about sex when what the migrant really needed was support with surviving in precarious circumstances.

We got much more bigger other problems … It's surviving first. … We [cannot] forget about the surviving and just sit there and think about HIV problems.

(Tony, Chinese gay man, aged 40)

For those who did attend support groups and found them useful, inter-dependence through shared common cultural values was more important than interdependence through sexual orientation.

STEPHEN: Starting from seven years ago I attended a group, Asian group, yum cha group. We get together and ... we talk and that's how – that's where I get most of the support and find out – find the places where I can get help. ...

INTERVIEWER: How important is it to you to have a group that consists of Asian people only?

STEPHEN: Very important. ... I get all my knowledge from there. And infor-mation about medicine, treatment and nutrition. ...

INTERVIEWER: ... How important is culture in this? Because you said it's very important that there are only Asians? ...

STEPHEN: Yes, important because Asians are more conservative and not as open as the Westerners. ... If you are all Asian or got the same cultural back-ground you can talk freely. There is no boundary in the culture. ... People [who] are from the same culture get together, then they can talk more comfortably.

(Stephen, Chinese gay man, aged 41)

## Cultural support

Almost all participants reported receiving one-on-one support from a bi-lingual MHAHS co-worker. This service is free at the point of access and available irrespective of migration status since no health care card is required. Such support made it possible for participants to behave independently and interdependently in different contexts across gender, sexual orientation and migration status. Bi-lingual co-workers assisted participants in behaving independently by providing language support and translation in dealing with social services and government agencies. As the co-workers are bound by a confidentiality agreement, participants were able to maintain interdependence with someone from the same culture and language without fearing disclosure.

[If there is] only one who I can tell everything ... I can talk in Thai – and he, I think that he signed that he cannot tell anyone else – then I tell everything.

(Som, Thai gay man, aged 33)

The co-workers gave some of the study participants an opportunity for inter-dependence by serving as a substitute for far-away family, from whom they did not have to conceal their HIV status and with whom there was no fear of rejection.

INTERVIEWER:  How long have you been with [co-worker]?

CHAMPEI:  Long time. Maybe '98 or something.

CO-WORKER:  Yes. She call me like a mum. ... The children call me grandma. (both laughing)

(Champei, Cambodian woman, aged 33)


## Discussion

In modern Western health care systems, and in order to provide the best possible outcomes, individuals are expected to make decisions about their own health. There are considerable obstacles to such independence and autonomy for migrants, however, especially for new migrants. These include legal status, an unfamiliar service landscape, lack of information, lack of social networks, and language difficulties, and they affect migrants across gender and sexual orientation. In this study, differences in service use across gender and sexual orientation were consistent with disclosure behaviour. No woman had disclosed her serostatus to anyone outside the health system. Women's decisions not to disclose were motivated by collectivist notions of interdependence and self-reliance (Körner 2007c). Similarly, women's use of health and social services was motivated by their relation to family and ethnic community: they limited their use of services to those necessary to maintain health and ensure survival in order to reduce the possibility of disclosure. In addition, women's pathways to, and use of, services were generally driven by others (Takahashi and Rodriguez 2002).

Heterosexual men positioned themselves as independent selves in their use of health and social services when they made decisions about what was best for them. For some, drawing on individualism and the independent self, not using social services meant living a normal life without being reminded of HIV. The collectivist orientation to interdependence was a motivation for heterosexual men with young children to seek services to look after their children when they themselves were no longer able to do so. The collectivist orientation also came into play when men avoided social services in order to protect their children from possible discrimination because of their father's HIV status (Körner 2007c).

Gay men positioned themselves in relation to individualist or collectivist cultural norms in different contexts and for different reasons. Similarly to women and heterosexual men with young children, interdependence with family might mean that some gay men went without social services in order to avoid disclosure and to protect the family's reputation. Unlike the women and like some heterosexual men, however, gay men positioned themselves independently in contexts that did not involve the family, where they were free to act according to their own wishes. Thus, rather than being a source of tension and conflict, collectivist and individualist values complemented each other. Gay men could take care of the collectivist needs of the family and at the same time of their individual needs separate from those of the family.

Interdependence with the gay community was more of a problem for some gay men. Welfare organizations and services for HIV-positive people in Australia were established by gay men, and predominantly for gay men. However, the Anglo-Celtic gay communities do not necessarily understand the more conservative cultural values of Asian gay men (Mao *et al.* 2002), nor do they meet the survival needs of migrant gay men (Keogh *et al.* 2004). In addition, Asian gay men are often marginalized in gay communities on racial grounds (Nemoto *et al.* 2003). For HIV-positive gay men from minority ethnic backgrounds, ethnicity can often be a more powerful uniting force than sexual orientation.

Gay men from ethnic minority communities may face problems in dealing with being both gay and belonging to an ethnic minority (Mao *et al.* 2002). This may be due to the tension between the individualist orientation of Western European cultures and the collectivist orientation of many Asian, South American and Southern European cultures, where family responsibilities and harmonious relationships with the kinship group are prioritized over individual desires. This tension is not easily resolved. Gay men from minority ethnic backgrounds need to manage their gay identity within their ethnic identities. Because of differing values they often feel alienated in mainstream gay communities (Peacock *et al.* 2001). At the same time, while social and cultural values of ethnic minorities are often hostile towards homosexuality, these values provide gay men with a sense of place and belonging in societies that are often racist (Keogh *et al.*, 2004).

## Conclusion

Rational models of health promotion are grounded in an individualist cultural orientation in which an independent, autonomous, informed and rational actor weighs costs and benefits in order to obtain the maximum benefit. For people from collectivist cultural backgrounds, however, decisions about health care and social services are located in a broader context of family and community, where social and cultural roles may prevent individuals from using health and social services in order to maintain interdependence with family and community (Bhattacharya 2004). Measures for health promotion, as well as for providing care and support, must thus include communities and their cultural values. Consideration also needs to be given not only to the material circumstances of migrants in general, but also to the social and cultural norms of different groups of migrants, such as gay men, heterosexual men, and women.

The response of minority ethnic communities to HIV has been dramatically different from the response of the gay community. In Australia, HIV services are embedded in the collective social and cultural lives of gay men: knowledge and use of such services is an integral part of gay life (Reid 2000; Takahashi and Rodriguez 2002). The same connection between HIV services and their social and cultural lives does not exist for HIV-positive people from minority ethnic groups.

Bi-lingual health workers serve as one way to bridge the gap between individuals from collectivist cultural backgrounds and health and social services in a predominantly individualist society. In this study, the MHAHS co-workers were essential to clinical support for people from minority backgrounds, for example by giving information about health and services, and by helping during doctors' appointments. Since they are bound by the laws and penalties that apply to all health workers in Australia, privacy and confidentiality are assured as the co-workers provide emotional and practical support.

In order to provide culturally appropriate care, health and social service workers in a society with a predominantly individualist orientation need better understanding of the self-in-relation-to-other of clients from societies with a predominantly collectivist orientation. At the same time, HIV-positive people from societies with a predominantly collectivist orientation, but living in countries which focus on the individual, need to be empowered to enable them to better utilize the choices offered within the health care system. Bi-lingual, bi-cultural, health workers are in a good position to bridge this gap. They act as brokers between individuals from ethnic minorities and the institutions of the individualist mainstream culture through the English language support they give, and by forming a link to ethnic communities through the mother tongue and shared cultural values.

## Notes

1 To ensure anonymity, all names have been changed.

## References

Anderson, J. and Doyal, L. (2004) 'Women from Africa living with HIV in London: a descriptive study', *AIDS Care*, *16*(1): 95–105.

Anderson, J. M., Wiggins, S., Rajwani, R., Holbrook, A., Blue, C. and Ng, M. (1995) 'Living with a chronic illness: Chinese-Canadian and Euro-Canadian women with diabetes – exploring factors that influence management', *Social Science & Medicine*, *41*(2): 181–95.

Bhattacharya, G. (2004) 'Health care seeking for HIV/AIDS among South Asians in the United States', *Health and Social Work*, *29*(2): 106–16.

Chin, D. and Kroesen, K. W. (1999) 'Disclosure of HIV infection among Asian/Pacific Islander American women: cultural stigma and support', *Cultural Diversity and Ethnic Minority Psychology*, *5*(3): 222–35.

Dore, G., Yueming, L., McDonald, A. and Kaldor, J. (2001) 'Spectrum of AIDS-defining illnesses in Australia 1992–98: influence of country/region of birth', *Journal of AIDS and Infectious Diseases*, *26*: 283–90.

Doyal, L. and Anderson, J. (2006) 'HIV-positive African women surviving in London: report of a qualitative study', *Gender and Development*, *14*(1): 95–104.

Epstein, S. (1995) 'The construction of lay experience: AIDS activism and the forging of credibility in the reform of clinical trials', *Science, Technology and Human Values*, *20*(4): 408–37.

Fogarty, A., Mao, L., Zablotska, I., Salter, M., Santana, H., Prestage, G., Rule, J., Canavan, P., Murphy, D. and McGuigan, D. (2006) *The Health in Men and Positive Health Cohorts. A Comparison of Trends in the Health and Sexual Behaviour of HIV-negative and HIV-positive Men, 2002–2005 (Monograph)*, Sydney: National Centre in HIV Social Research, University of New South Wales.

Fogarty, A., Rawstorne, P., Prestage, G., Grierson, J., Grulich, A., Kippax, S., Worth, H. and Murphy, D. (2003) *Positive Health: Then and Now – Following HIV-positive People's Lives Over Time (Monograph)*, Sydney: National Centre in HIV Social Research, University of New South Wales.

Holman, H. and Lorig, K. (2000) 'Patients as partners in managing chronic disease', *British Medical Journal, 320*: 526–27.

Ishikawa, H. and Yamazaki, Y. (2005) 'How applicable are western models of patient-physician relationships in Asia? Changing patient-physician relationship in contemporary Japan', *International Journal of Japanese Sociology, 14*: 84–93.

Jorgensen, M. J. and Marwit, S. J. (2001) 'Emotional support needs of gay males with AIDS', *AIDS Care, 13*(2): 171–75.

Keogh, P., Dodds, C. and Henderson, L. (2004) *Migrant Gay Men: Redefining Community, Restoring Identity*, London: Sigma Research.

Kitayama, S., Markus, H. R., Matsumoto, H. and Norasakkunkit, V. (1997) 'Individual and collective processes in the construction of the self: self-enhancement in the United States and self-criticism in Japan', *Journal of Personality and Social Psychology, 72*(6): 1245–67.

Körner, H. (2007a) 'Late HIV diagnosis of people from culturally and linguistically diverse backgrounds in Sydney: the role of culture and community', *AIDS Care, 19*(2): 168–78.

—— (2007b) '"If I had my residency I wouldn't worry": negotiating migration and HIV in Sydney, Australia', *Ethnicity & Health, 12*(3): 205–25.

—— (2007c) 'Negotiating cultures: disclosure of HIV-positive status among people from ethnic minorities in Sydney', *Culture, Health and Sexuality, 9*(2): 137–52.

Leong, F. T. L. and Lau, A. S. L. (2001) 'Barriers to providing effective mental health services to Asian Americans', *Mental Health Services Research, 3*(4): 201–14.

Mao, L., McCormick, J. and Van De Ven, P. (2002) 'Ethnic and gay identification: gay Asian men dealing with the divide', *Culture, Health and Sexuality, 4*(4): 419–30.

Mao, L., Van De Ven, P., Prestage, G., Wang, J., Hua, M., Prihaswan, P. and Ku, A. (2003) *Asian Gay Community Periodic Survey Sydney 2002 (Monograph)*, Sydney: National Centre in HIV Social Research, University of New South Wales.

Marelich, W. D., Johnston Roberts, K., Murphy, D. A. and Callari, T. (2002) 'HIV/AIDS patient involvement in antiretroviral treatment decisions', *AIDS Care, 14*(1): 17–26.

Markus, H. R. and Kitayama, S. (1991) 'Culture and the self: implications for cognition, emotion and motivation', *Psychological Review, 98*(2): 224–53.

—— (1994) 'A collective fear of the collective: implications for selves and theories of selves', *Personality and Social Psychology Bulletin, 20*(5): 568–79.

McDonald, A., Yueming, L. and Dore, G. J. (2003) 'Late HIV presentation among AIDS cases in Australia, 1992–2001', *Australian and New Zealand Journal of Public Health, 27*(6): 608–13.

Mead, N. and Bower, P. (2000) 'Patient-centredness: a conceptual framework and review of the empirical literature', *Social Science & Medicine, 51*: 1087–110.

Nemoto, T., Operario, D., Soma, T., Bao, D., Vajrabukka, A. and Crisostomo, V. (2003) 'HIV risk and prevention among Asian/Pacific Islander men who have sex with men: listen to our stories', *AIDS Education and Prevention, 15*(Supplement A): 7–20.

Peacock, B., Eyre, S. L., Quinn, S. C. and Kegeles, S. (2001) 'Delineating differences: sub-communities in the San Francisco gay community', *Culture, Health and Sexuality, 2001*(3): 183–201.

Persson, A., Barton, D. and Richards, W. (2006) *Men and Women Living Heterosexually with HIV. The Straightpoz Study, Volume 1 (Monograph)*, Sydney: National Centre in HIV Social Research, University of New South Wales.

Reid, P. T. (2000) 'Women, ethnicity and AIDS: what's love got to do with it?', *Sex Roles, 7*(8): 709–22.

Shedlin, M. G. and Shulman, L. (2004) 'Qualitative needs assessment of HIV services among Dominican, Mexican and Central American immigrant populations living in the New York City area', *AIDS Care, 16*(4): 434–45.

Takahashi, L. M. and Rodriguez, R. (2002) 'Access redefined: service pathways of persons living with HIV and AIDS', *Culture, Health and Sexuality, 4*(1): 67–83.

Triandis, H. C. (1989) 'The self and social behavior in differing cultural contexts', *Psychological Review, 96*(3): 506–20.

—— (1995) *Individualism and Collectivism*, Boulder, Colorado: Westview Press.

Triandis, H. C., Bontempo, R., Vallareal, M. J., Asai, M. and Lucca, N. (1988) 'Individualism and collectivism: cross-cultural perspectives on self–ingroup relationships', *Journal of Personality and Social Psychology, 54*(2): 323–38.

# Chapter 6

# Treat with care

## Africans and HIV in the UK

*Jane Anderson*

The current era of global population movement, together with longstanding historical and political relationships between many nations in Africa and those in Western Europe means that more people are travelling to and from countries with high rates of HIV infection than ever before. This in turn is influencing the epidemiology of HIV infection and care in Europe (Hamers and Downs 2004). In England, the prevalence of diagnosed HIV in communities of black African origin is estimated to be 3.7 per cent compared to 0.09 per cent among the white population. Data from the Health Protection Agency (2008) suggest that a majority of these infections are in heterosexuals and have mainly been acquired in countries in Africa. In total, 24,800 people born in sub-Saharan Africa were living with HIV in the UK in 2006. Many others remained undiagnosed and unaware of their infection (UK Collaborative Group for HIV and STI Surveillance 2007).

Despite these statistics, the body of knowledge about the ways that HIV affects the lives of Africans in the UK diasporas remains limited. Yet such under-standings are of fundamental importance for the successful design and imple-mentation of health care responses for HIV prevention, diagnosis and treatment. This chapter examines some of the experiences facing HIV-positive African migrants seeking treatment and care in the UK. A number of shared experiences have been reported amongst members of this group, particularly regarding treatment access. However, after examining the wider context within which migrants can seek HIV treatment, the chapter also draws out some of the dif-ferences in the lived experiences faced by (self-defined) heterosexual women, heterosexual men and gay/bisexual men in accessing care and building a life within the UK.

The chapter is informed by current literature and by data obtained from four research studies in which the author has been involved over the past decade in specialist HIV clinical services in London. One was a large-scale quantitative survey (cf. Elford *et al.* 2006), and three were qualitative projects (cf. Anderson and Doyal 2004; Doyal and Anderson 2005; Doyal *et al.* 2005; Paparini *et al.* 2008). Access to HIV patient populations was enabled by the author's work as a clinician in this field.

## Asylum, health care and treatment eligibility

For some people, the decision to migrate from Africa to the UK will be voluntary, whilst others will face situations in which they are forced to leave home. Either way, negotiating a new culture, different health care systems and other ways of living are part of the process for all. Many Africans arriving in the UK are unaware of their HIV status, only discovering their diagnosis some years later, thus refuting popular media reports of 'HIV treatment tourism' (National AIDS Trust 2008). Nonetheless, although rarely a reason why people leave 'home', HIV and its treatment may be one of the underlying reasons some people wish to secure a future in the UK. Particular challenges face those who are applicants for asylum, many of whom may have a history of serious trauma, torture or conflict which engenders additional vulnerability and health care needs. Asylum applicants are often portrayed as 'undeserving' and separate from 'genuine' refugees (Sales 2002), thus being both an asylum applicant and living with HIV means carrying a doubly compromised social identity (Dodds *et al.* 2004). High levels of poverty and destitution have been described amongst asylum applicants, exacerbated by their inability to work in the UK whilst their case is being considered. The geographical dispersal of asylum applicants and cases of refused applicants being detained, further complicate good HIV clinical care (Creighton *et al.* 2004).

For those who are refused asylum, removal from the UK may mean that people are returned to parts of the world with minimal or no access to HIV care. Even for those allowed to stay in the UK, uncertainty over their future frequently persists and pervades their experiences of health and wellbeing. Despite, in 2005, the British Government playing a lead role in the global pledge to ensure universal access to HIV treatment prevention and care by 2010, UK domestic policy initiatives have been devised in a climate where the connections between HIV/AIDS, asylum and migration were becoming increasingly problematic, with reactionary and frequently hostile media coverage (Ingram 2008). In response, the regulations for free National Health Service (NHS) care for overseas visitors were revised, reducing or withdrawing access to HIV treatment and care for certain people in England and Wales, despite the UK commitment to global universal access through the United Nations (UN) agreement. At the same time, rulings in the English courts led to the removal of people living with HIV from the UK to parts of the world with still far from adequate provision of HIV treatment and care. Although various easement clauses have been introduced more recently (e.g. permitting ongoing free HIV care for those with failed asylum applications if treatment was begun before the application outcome), considerable confusion exists within health services and charges may still be applied in situations where care should be free.

### 'Black Africans' and HIV in the UK

The use of the term 'Black African' as a descriptive category for people living with HIV in the UK gives the impression of a homogeneous population group.

This is far from the case and, despite a variety of shared attributes, this form of categorisation masks significant areas of diversity (Agyemang *et al.* 2005; Aspinall and Chinouya 2008). The African diasporas in the UK include newly arrived migrants as well as established, settled communities living away from Africa over several generations. This means that experiences of living with HIV are diverse, even within the same communities and geographical locations. Many factors affect the ways in which HIV is played out in real lives. Both gender and sexual identity are important here and are complicated by multiple structural, political, cultural and social influences which impact on the ways in which illness is experienced.

Despite these differences, studies of Africans and HIV in the UK reveal some common themes (cf. Green and Smith 2004; Prost *et al.* 2008). Data on HIV-related deaths in the UK show that the majority now occur in those who do not access diagnosis and treatment early enough (Lucas *et al.* 2008). Despite recent health promotion efforts and developments in therapy, Africans, particularly men and those who have been in the UK for shorter periods of time, consistently present later to HIV services than British-born people (Chadborn *et al.* 2006). A compounding factor in late diagnosis is the imperfect awareness of HIV risk by UK clinicians. Data show that many migrants access health care services, but practitioners frequently do not use these encounters to address HIV or offer testing (Burns *et al.* 2008). In addition, many African people in the UK do not consider themselves to be at personal risk, particularly if they feel well and are in a regular relationship (Dodds *et al.* 2008). Many may have witnessed the ill health and death associated with untreated HIV in a 'home' setting and may be unaware of efficacious treatment. The stigma associated with HIV within many African communities leads to fear of discrimination and potential rejection (Calin *et al.* 2007; Elford *et al.* 2008a). This in turn is closely associated with anxieties about confidentiality of information and problems of disclosure to other people. For many, health services may not be easy to negotiate, language may present a problem, eligibility for appropriate care if found to be infected and health beliefs will all have an impact. Life is often complex and beset with other more immediate survival and psychosocial issues, lowering the priority for health care.

Despite the partially unifying effect of these overarching issues, the diversity of lived experience of HIV remains, with factors of gender, sexual identity and sexual lifestyles playing important roles. Making sense of how these variable factors intersect with one another in shaping the experiences of individuals living with and responding to HIV is critically important if relevant and effective programmes and interventions are to be found (Doyal 2009).

## Gender, sexual orientation, HIV and health care

Sexuality and ethnicity as they relate to HIV in the UK are tightly linked. Most Africans living with HIV in the UK are heterosexual, and the majority of heterosexuals living with HIV are of African origin. By contrast, the majority of white, British-born people with HIV are gay men (UK Collaborative Group for HIV and STI Surveillance 2007). Consequently, much of the UK-based understanding of how heterosexual men and women experience HIV is derived from work with people of African origin whilst the needs and experiences of African men with HIV who have sex with men have been largely overlooked or assumed to not exist (Doyal *et al.* 2008; Paparini *et al.* 2008).

Despite the central role of sex and gender in the aetiology of HIV, little data exist to help understand the impact in the experiences and management of HIV in African communities in the UK. Interventions to prevent onward transmission of HIV rely heavily on the negotiation of safer sexual practices such as condom use. However, African heterosexual women with HIV in the UK, describe not only a lack of power in these negotiations with men but also issues of non-consenting sex and the possibility that being assertive might result in violence (Ridge *et al.* 2007).

Data from studies undertaken amongst African people living with HIV in London provide some insights into the ways in which sexuality and gender may impact on HIV and vice versa in this population. During 2004–5 a questionnaire survey of almost 1,700 HIV-positive hospital attendees was carried out across six HIV specialist NHS clinics (cf. Elford *et al.* 2006). The study enrolled adults with diagnosed HIV who gave written informed consent and returned a completed questionnaire (response rate 73 per cent of eligible clinic attendees). This comprised 480 black African heterosexual women, 224 black African heterosexual men and 758 gay/bisexual men (a majority, 464 white). Only 13 African men identifying themselves as gay/bisexual were enrolled, making it difficult to draw any meaningful conclusions about this group.

Analysis was based on the two largest population groups, namely gay men (mostly white) and African heterosexual men and women. It is important to acknowledge that there were many shared characteristics despite this dividing line. Experiences of HIV stigma and discrimination were reported across both populations as were high levels of poverty and deprivation. Although higher for African respondents, a significant number of white gay men were living in difficult financial circumstances, highlighting the increasing association of HIV with poverty within the UK (Ibrahim *et al.* 2008).

Information obtained about sexual behaviour suggests that heterosexual African people with HIV in London are less likely to report sexual activity that presents a risk of onward transmission to sexual partners than gay men. One in five of the gay men with HIV reported unprotected anal intercourse with a partner of unknown or discordant HIV status. In comparison, one in 20 black African heterosexual men and women reported unprotected vaginal intercourse that presented a risk of HIV transmission. Most black Africans reported unprotected intercourse with a main partner rather than a casual partner, and the men were more likely to report unprotected intercourse with a main partner who was HIV positive (9.8 per cent) than a partner who was HIV negative or of unknown HIV status (2.1 per cent).

Rates of disclosure of HIV status to a sexual partner were lower amongst black Africans, with heterosexual women having the lowest rates of disclosure (Elford *et al.* 2008b). Further data from this study confirmed the central importance of religious beliefs for African heterosexuals, particularly women, with HIV, and their social and economic circumstances were significantly less satisfactory than those of HIV-positive mostly white gay men (Ibrahim *et al.* 2008).

Three qualitative studies focusing on the experiences of (self-defined) African heterosexual women (Anderson and Doyal 2004; Doyal and Anderson 2005), African heterosexual men (Doyal *et al.* 2005) and African men who have sex with other men (Paparini *et al.* 2008), all living with HIV, were also undertaken between 2001 and 2006. All studies drew upon in-depth semi-structured interviews to examine the experience of HIV infection in the broader context of the individuals' life history and current circumstances.

All participants had been born in Africa, and had lived in the UK and been diagnosed with HIV for at least six months. Sample sizes reflected the difficulties involved in recruiting subjects in each group, with African gay men being especially hard to reach. However, the eventual samples matched the sizes of the different groups in the overall population of black Africans living with HIV in the UK. The first study included 62 heterosexual women, the second 45 heterosexual men and the third eight African gay/bisexual men. Migration stage, the process of immigration, HIV-associated stigma and discrimination (real and perceived), problems associated with disclosure and confidentiality, social and sexual relationships and the day-to-day complexities of life were consistent themes across all three studies.

For many people, HIV health care services and specialist professionals were seen to be a source of support and the clinical environment was the only place where HIV could be discussed fully. The sometimes complex drug regimens that were involved in treatment was an issue. For some whose family and friends were often far away, returning to them would compromise access to medication, with some people describing themselves as 'trapped' by the treatment. However, there were also differences in the experiences of HIV between the three groups.

### Heterosexual women

The shock of the diagnosis reverberated throughout the interviews of this group. In particular, women who were married or who had few sexual partners did not feel they 'fitted' the imagined model of the HIV-positive person. As one woman explained, 'I didn't have any cause to think about that. I was such a lady, I would never have thought of that'. Those who had been found to be HIV positive because of the ill health or death of a partner or child had to deal with notions of guilt, betrayal and bereavement as well as their own diagnosis. Family and the centrality of the woman's role within it was a defining theme in women's experiences of living with HIV. As one woman put it,

It's like your responsibility as the mother to keep the family together. ... No matter what the man is doing, no matter what's happening, whether he's supporting you financially or morally or otherwise, you know, you just have to try and keep the family together.

(Nigerian woman, 35 years old)[1]

Existing children, both those in the UK and those who were separated geographically were of fundamental importance. Women described the imperative to remain in good health both to care for children and to remain financially viable to provide for them materially. Women whose children were living away from them described the tension between being separated from their children and yet having access to health care in London which, in the longer term, would allow them to support their families for greater periods of time. The link between pregnancy and a first HIV diagnosis in the context of routine antenatal HIV screening programmes gave women's experience of HIV a particular poignancy, with concerns about passing HIV to their children, and the relief they experienced when a child was found to be uninfected.

The same issues about transmission to others coloured women's sexual relationships and future child-bearing intentions, many expressing a wish for more children but perceiving risks to both partners and unborn children. Describing the risks of attempting to conceive another child one woman explained, 'We won't try to do it without any protection, it's bad enough I'm HIV positive, I can't risk my husband becoming positive as well' (Nigerian woman, 35 years old).

Women talked about the risks of disclosure of an HIV diagnosis to other family members and the effects it would have, not only on the family structure but also the woman's place within it. They spoke of their fears of potential abandonment and of being disowned by partners and family. The issue of disclosure to a male partner is summed up in the words of one participant: 'It took me about 11 months before I told him. I had prepared myself in case he threw me out of the house' (Kenyan woman, 37 years old). The expectation of such responses was a major factor for women who had yet to disclose, and information management in general was a key feature of a life lived with HIV. Sisters would often be told before parents and telling children was considered particularly difficult with its underlying implication of parental sexuality. Religious belief was one of the strongest supports for women and both organised religion and private prayer were seen as central to getting through life with HIV. As one woman said:

I had to rely on God, only God, and I just used to pray to God every time, and I said, God all I ask you is please give the doctors wisdom, let them find some medicine in future. And I just had the strong belief that there would come, that one day there would be some medicine, and I said keep me alive until that time.

(Ugandan woman, 39 years old)

### Heterosexual men

For many African men, the experience of HIV in the UK was associated with loss, weakness and loneliness. As one man said, 'When you are HIV positive you are not as strong as you used to be, so you can be a man but you are weak' (Ugandan man, 44 years old). They lost not only physical health and well being, but also future hopes and ambitions, plans for relationships and for fatherhood. Meeting their own expectations as well as those of the wider community whilst coping with HIV was a challenge described by many. The sense of unfulfilled aspirations was summed up by one man who stated,

> There's a lot I really wanted to do. There's a lot I wanted to prove. I just don't have the motivation within me anymore. I just don't have it now. I wonder what has happened to that person that I was when I first came to this country. My life has been shattered.
>
> (Malawian man, 29 years old)

The lack of financial independence resulting from their position as migrants and/or because of ill health compromised many men's sense of themselves even further, making them increasingly dependent on others. This, in turn, had the potential to disrupt the balance of power between the men and their female partners and to damage relationships. Indeed, the idea of forming lasting relationships with women was compromised by HIV, both because of possible risks of onward transmission to partners and ideas about how women might respond to them. As one respondent explained, 'I don't socialise. If I see a girl is interested in me I just keep away, I don't lead them on now; I brush them aside because I know what I have got' (Zimbabwean man, 39 years old). Most men described a significant reduction in sexual activity following their diagnosis of HIV, even with regular partners, one man describing his experience saying, 'I can't even enjoy sex with my wife. ... Sex comes from the mind, if you have a free mind, so I'm not free therefore I cannot enjoy sex. So that's why' (Rwandan, 40 years old).

The desire for children was expressed by many men, but as something that was seen as less likely to happen for them during a life lived with HIV. Disclosure of HIV status to others was a particular issue, although most of those interviewed had told regular sexual partners of their infection. Telling parents was especially challenging, often because they were far away and because the impact of the potential loss of a son was felt to be too great a burden to inflict. These factors taken together reduced the quantity and quality of social relationships, which culminated in feelings of isolation, loneliness and powerlessness.

Although important, religious belief played a smaller role in the lives of the heterosexual men than of the women. Finding employment and remaining well enough to work and earn a living was the most important aim for many men and was viewed as a key to survival and their future well being. At the same time, men described the importance of making the most of whatever time they had and taking responsibility for improving their situation. On a positive note echoed by several other men, one man commented about the future, saying:

> I am hopeful. Something better for all of us. I am going to be around for quite a long while now. How everything is going to come out at the end of the day, we'll see when I get there.
>
> (Zimbabwean man, 35 years old)

### Gay men

The complicated nature of keeping life intact as an African gay man living with HIV in the UK was repeatedly emphasised. The key to this process appeared for a majority to lie in withholding aspects of their lives and identities from other people, resulting in very restricted opportunities for men to be fully themselves. Talking about disclosure, one man explained:

> No, I haven't told anyone, I've never told them ... because it will destroy the family and I don't think they will be able to cope with it ... And I think they would distance themselves completely away from me ... it's bad enough me being gay, and if they found out that I'm HIV I don't think they will give in ... they will find it very difficult for me to be around them, I think, anyway.[2]

As both HIV and homosexuality remain stigmatised issues in many African communities (Doyal *et al.* 2008) the men found themselves carrying a double burden, with their position as migrants within the wider community adding a further layer of complexity to their lives. Relative to being in Africa, attitudes to homosexual relationships in London provided a freedom of expression that few had encountered before arriving in the UK, but relationships in that environment were largely with non-African people. Spaces in which men could be openly African *and* gay were very hard to find. In particular, HIV-specific support mechanisms were either focused towards heterosexual Africans or towards British-born gay men making them difficult for African gay men to negotiate.

Once again, for members of this group, the importance of family and children came to the fore, as men described the importance of having children and the centrality of relationships with parents and family members. The importance of having children, either with female partners or through adoption with same-sex partners was highlighted by many. As one man put it,

> It's just my way. All my brothers, or cousins, have children and in African way, you have to have children, what's wrong with you, if you don't have

children? It's not that I want to have children because someone wants me to have children. ... it's just because I want to be a father and I want to have a child, and love him, or her, and give him, or her, my love and know that I have a child ...

Religious belief was a particularly difficult issue for this group of men and a source of tension and ambivalence. Although all believed in the existence of God and saw their faith as a source of support, many felt that the teachings and atmosphere of organised religious gatherings were particularly unsympathetic to homosexuality and avoided them, as summed up by one respondent:

I felt very guilty for a long time, being gay I was very confused ... Now since I'm bigger, since I got older, religion is important to me. I pray to God, but I find it very guilty when I go to church being gay, positive.

## Conclusions

A gap remains between recent biomedical advances in the management of HIV and their translation into reality for those infected. Despite wide geographical variations in the affordability and availability of sophisticated monitoring and antiretroviral therapy across the world, inequalities remain even in the world's richest nations. Asylum seekers, refugees and undocumented migrants are often amongst the most vulnerable in society, and are likely to have the least power to obtain what they need in terms of health care. The high levels of late presentation amongst African people with HIV compromise the long-term benefits that can be achieved with antiretroviral agents. Initiatives to encourage earlier diagnosis and increase testing for HIV, however, must be feasible for people who have many other challenges in life and for whom treatment may not even be freely available within the NHS. HIV-associated stigma, both real and anticipated, continues to have a paralysing effect on communities and individuals of African origin within the UK. However, the potential clinical benefits of being in the UK are well recognised by Africans with HIV and the specialist clinical services, once accessed, are appreciated and valued.

The particular ways in which individuals deal with HIV are significantly influenced by gender and sexuality and these must be key considerations for those planning and delivering HIV-related prevention and direct health care in the UK. The central role of family is clear and yet how to sustain and provide for that family and how to be fully oneself within the family in the face of HIV infection remains a central challenge. Understanding the impact that HIV has on one's ability to be a 'proper' woman, to be a 'strong' man and, especially difficult, to uphold an identity as a gay/bisexual African man is crucial to providing the most relevant treatment and care.

## Acknowledgements

The people who took part in the studies described here have shared complex and difficult stories with the research teams and I hope we have represented adequately the lives we have been privileged to study. Lesley Doyal was instrumental in the design and analysis of the three qualitative studies. Jonathan Elford played a major role in the quantitative study. Patricia Apenteng, Cecelia Bukutu, Fowzia Ibrahim and Sara Paparini all helped with data collection, analysis and writing. We were consistently supported by a wide range of voluntary sector organisations and by individuals who informed the research questions and process.

## Notes

1 Names are not given in order to protect participant identity.
2 The voices of the men are represented using quotes from their narratives. However, because of the very small sample size, no identifying data are provided here.

## References

Agyemang, C., Bhopal, R. and Bruijnzeels, M. (2005) 'Negro, Black, Black African, African Caribbean, African American or what? Labelling African origin populations in the health arena in the 21st century', *Journal of Epidemiology and Community Health*, 59: 1014–18.

Anderson, J. and Doyal, L. (2004) 'Women from Africa living with HIV in London: a descriptive study', *AIDS Care*, 16: 95–105.

Aspinall, J. and Chinouya, M. (2008) 'Is the standardised term "Black African" useful in demographic and health research in the United Kingdom?', *Ethnicity & Health*, 13: 183–202.

Burns, F. M., Johnson, A. M., Nazroo, J., Ainsworth, J., Anderson, J., Fakoya, A., Fakoya, I., Hughes, A., Jungmann, E., Sadiq, S. T., Sullivan, A. K. and Fenton, K. A. (2008) 'Missed opportunities for earlier HIV diagnosis within primary and secondary healthcare settings in the UK', *AIDS*, 22: 115–22.

Calin, T., Green, J., Hetherton, J. and Brook, G. (2007) 'Disclosure of HIV among Black African men and women attending a London HIV clinic', *AIDS Care*, 19(3): 385–91.

Chadborn, T. R., Delpech, V. C., Sabin, C. A., Sinka, K. and Evans, B. G. (2006) 'The late diagnosis and consequent short-term mortality of HIV-infected heterosexuals (England and Wales, 2000–2004)', *AIDS*, 20: 2371–79.

Creighton, S., Sethi, G., Edwards, S. G. and Miller, R. (2004) 'Dispersal of HIV positive asylum seekers: national survey of UK healthcare providers', *British Medical Journal*, 329: 322–23.

Dodds, C., Hickson, F., Weatherburn, P., Reid, D., Hammond, G., Jessup, K. and Adegbite, G. (2008) *BASS Line 2007 Survey. Assessing the Sexual HIV Prevention Needs of African People in England*. London: Sigma Research.

Dodds, C., Keogh, K., Chime, O., Haruperi, T., Nabulya, B., Ssanya Sseruma, W. and Weatherburn, P. (2004) *Outsider Status: Stigma and Discrimination Experienced by Gay Men and African People with HIV*. London: Sigma Research.

Doyal, L. (2009) 'Challenges in researching life with HIV and AIDS: an intersectional analysis of black African migrants in London', *Culture, Health and Sexuality*, 11(2): 173–88.

Doyal, L. and Anderson, J. (2005) '"My fear is to fall in love again … " how HIV-positive African women survive in London', *Social Science & Medicine*, 60: 1729–38.

Doyal, L., Anderson, J. and Apenteng, P. (2005) *'I Want to Survive, I Want to Win, I Want Tomorrow': An Exploratory Study of African Men Living with HIV in London*. London: Homerton University Hospital NHS Foundation Trust.

Doyal, L., Paparini, S. and Anderson, J. (2008) '"Elvis died and I was born": black African Men negotiating same-sex desire in London', *Sexualities*, 11: 171–92.

Elford, J., Anderson, J., Bukutu, C. and Ibrahim, F. (2006) 'HIV in East London: ethnicity, gender and risk. Design and methods', *BMC Public Health*, 6: 150.

Elford, J., Ibrahim, F., Bukutu, C. and Anderson, J. (2008a) 'HIV-related discrimination reported by people living with HIV in London, UK', *AIDS Behaviour*, 12: 255–64.

Elford, J., Ibrahm, F., Bukutu, C. and Anderson, J. (2008b) 'Disclosure of HIV status: the role of ethnicity among people living with HIV in London', *Journal of Acquired Immune Deficiency Syndrome*, 47: 514–21.

Green, G. and Smith, R. (2004) 'The psychosocial and health care needs of HIV-positive people in the United Kingdom: a review', *HIV Medicine*, 5: 5–46.

Hamers, F. F. and Downs, A. M. (2004) 'The changing face of the HIV epidemic in western Europe: what are the implications for public health policies?' *Lancet*, 364: 83–94.

Health Protection Agency (2008) *Sexually Transmitted Infections in Black African and Black Caribbean Communities in the UK: 2008 Report*. London: Health Protection Agency.

Ibrahim, F., Anderson, J., Bukutu, C. and Elford, J. (2008) 'Social and economical hardship among people living with HIV in London', *HIV Medicine*, 9: 616–24.

Ingram, A. (2008) 'Domopolitics and disease: HIV/AIDS, immigration, and asylum in the UK', *Environment and Planning D: Society and Space*, 26: 875–94.

Lucas, S. B., Curtis, H. and Johnson, M. A. (2008) 'National review of deaths among HIV-infected adults', *Clinical Medicine*, 8: 250–52.

National AIDS Trust (2008) *The Myth of HIV Health Tourism*. London: National AIDS Trust.

Paparini, S., Doyal, L. and Anderson, J. (2008) '"I count myself as being in a different world": African gay and bisexual men living with HIV in London. An exploratory study', *AIDS Care*, 20: 601–5.

Prost, A., Elford, J., Imrie, J., Petticrew, M. and Hart, G. J. (2008) 'Social, behavioural, and intervention research among people of Sub-Saharan African origin living with HIV in the UK and Europe: literature review and recommendations for intervention', *AIDS Behaviour*, 12: 170–94.

Ridge, D., Ziebalnd, S., Anderson, J., Williams, I. and Elford, J. (2007) 'Positive prevention: contemporary issues facing HIV positive people negotiating sex in the UK', *Social Science & Medicine*, 65: 755–70.

Sales, R. (2002) 'The deserving and the undeserving? Refugees, asylum seekers and welfare in Britain', *Critical Social Policy*, 22: 456–78.

UK Collaborative Group for HIV and STI Surveillance (2007) *Testing Times: HIV and Other Sexually Transmitted Infections in the United Kingdom*. London: Health Protection Agency, Centre for Infections.

# Chapter 7

# Touristic borderlands
## Ethnographic reflections on Dominican social geographies

*Mark B. Padilla and H. Daniel Castellanos*

This chapter draws on findings from ethnographic research among male sex workers in the Dominican Republic who work in the borderlands between globalized tourism areas and surrounding local communities. It takes as its point of departure the notion that experiences of globalization can be profoundly shaped by local or sub-national shifts in the social geography of space. When entry into particular social spaces comes to 'stand in' for global experiences, people may symbolically transport themselves into the 'global' arena through entry into these spaces. Further, we argue that these vicarious global experiences have a particular quality in tourism areas, where impoverished service workers who are functionally excluded from global mobility intermingle with a wide range of global 'elites', for whom such mobility is a taken-for-granted source of pride and modern social capital. Tourism areas are therefore particular kinds of borderlands between the local and the global, creating experiences that are bounded by geography and stark social hierarchies (localizing effects), while allowing for play and a temporary, partial escape from normative constraints as one 'opens up' to the global (globalizing effects).

These tensions between the localizing and globalizing effects of tourism areas have become more salient in the past few decades due to dramatic changes in Caribbean social geographies. As the tourism industry has become the primary economic driver of Caribbean economies, a growing proportion of local populations are making a marginal living by traversing the boundaries that separate two very different lived realities: those of foreigners who travel to coastal areas in search of sun and sand, and those of the local service providers who serve these temporary visitors. The touristic borderlands that form the terrain in which these two populations interact are often located within gated communities or spatially bounded areas characterized by strong social and economic inequalities; low wages and job insecurity for service providers; a diverse informal 'pleasure industry' that provides intimate services such as massage, hair braiding, cultural exchange, and sex; intense population mobility and mixing; and a cultural climate that is markedly distinct from other parts of the local or national environment (Padilla 2007a). We therefore define touristic borderlands as spaces with the localizing and globalizing characteristics described above, and which tend to exist as geographically separable terrains in which the logic, erotic climate, and instrumental rationality of the tourism industry pervade nearly all features of social life.

While global epidemiological research on HIV has shown consistent associations between migration and viral transmission (see, for example, Bronfman et al. 1989; Jochelson et al. 1991; Broring and Van Duifhuizen 1993; Decosas 1998; Benoît 1999), relatively little ethnographic work has been conducted to understand how migratory environments are understood or experienced as social spaces, a fact which reduces the relevance of much research for the design of meaningful programs or interventions. In addition, much existing research on HIV and migration neglects a consideration of tourism areas as particular kinds of destinations of labour migration, and the lack of such research is particularly pronounced in the Caribbean.

While a complete analysis of the characteristics of touristic borderlands is beyond the scope of this chapter, here we reflect on the social and sexual integration of touristic borderlands within the actual and fantasized travels of young Dominican male sex workers. In exploring how men encounter and experience these spaces, we draw upon ethnographic data derived from a larger anthropological research project led by the first author (Padilla 2007b). Data include ethnographic observations within social networks of male sex workers, in-depth interviews with 72 male sex workers, and an extensive demographic, behavioural and social survey with 200 sex workers. This chapter draws primarily on an analysis of the in-depth interviews. Data collection for these interviews occurred in 2001, and was assisted by the first author's affiliation with the Dominican non-governmental organization, *Amigos Siempre Amigos*, and involved snowball sampling male sex workers through a wide range of social networks that were identified through a first phase of the study. Table 7.1 summarizes the characteristics of the in-depth interview sample, by research site.

## Population mobility and the growth of 'tourism poles' in the Dominican Republic

In the last 50 years, the Dominican Republic has experienced a dramatic increase in population, growing from 3.8 million in 1960 to 8.9 million in 2005 (Lozano 1997; World Bank Development Data Group 2006). Over the same period, the country has also experienced the most significant population migration of its modern history, both from rural to urban/semi-urban areas and from the Dominican Republic to international destinations. In the case of national migration, the largest migration has been to the capital city of Santo Domingo, growing from half a million people, or 12 per cent of the total population, in 1960 (Lozano 1997) to 2.7 million people or 31 per cent of the total population in 2002 (Oficina Nacional de Estadística 2004).

After migrating to urban settings, a large number of Dominican families face a new labour market. Lacking adequate education and job skills, migrants often

*Table 7.1* Characteristics of interview sample, by research site (N=72)

| | % (n) | |
| --- | --- | --- |
| | Santo Domingo (n=42)[a] | Boca Chica (n=23)[a] |
| Age (years) | Mean age=24.8 | Mean age=26.1 |
| 18–20 | 26.2 (11) | 26.0 (6) |
| 21–25 | 28.6 (12) | 21.7 (5) |
| 26–30 | 21.4 (9) | 26.1 (6) |
| 31–35 | 11.9 (5) | 17.4 (4) |
| >36 | 4.8 (2) | 4.3 (1) |
| No response | 7.1 (3) | 4.3 (1) |
| % with at least one stable partner | 59.5 (25) | 39.1 (9) |
| % of above whose stable partner(s) are male | 20.0 (5) | 11.1 (1) |
| % of above whose stable partner(s) are female | 48.0 (12) | 66.7 (6) |
| % of above whose stable partners are of both sexes | 32.0 (8) | 22.2 (2) |
| % living with family members | 71.4 (30) | 56.5 (13) |
| % married | 29.0 (12) | 8.7 (2) |
| % with children | 45.2 (19) | 60.9 (14) |

[a] Sociodemographic data unavailable for 7 interviewees (4 in Santo Domingo, 3 in Boca Chica)

depend on the informal urban economy as the primary source of income (Lozano 1997). These household-level economic changes and the extensive rural-to-urban migration have not only depopulated rural areas and dislocated existing family and support networks, but have also overburdened the receiving urban settings, which have seen drastic increases in unemployment, homelessness, and poverty (Morel and Mejía 1996; Lozano 1997).

In addition to this population transition from rural to urban areas, a considerable number of Dominicans have migrated to the USA and Europe. Estimates of the number of Dominican immigrants currently in the USA vary widely, with some as high as a million (Georges 1990). More conservative estimates are closer to a half million, or equivalent to 6 per cent of the population of the Dominican Republic itself (Grasmuck and Pessar 1991). Tourism and family visits to the USA are now a fact of life for many middle-class Dominicans, and among Santo Domingo residents it is very common to have at least one extended family member who resides abroad. 'Dominicanyorks', a term used to describe Dominicans residing for significant periods in New York City, have come to symbolize the contemporary reality that Dominican national identity now straddles two very different islands: Hispaniola and Manhattan.

In the last few decades, the country has also seen new migratory patterns resulting from the rise of tourism. Unlike other Central and South American countries such as Costa Rica, Mexico, or Brazil, tourism in the Dominican

Republic has been primarily organized around what the Dominican government calls *polos turísticos* or tourism poles. By investing in infrastructure and inviting multinational investment within these poles, the country's development experts hoped to foster a 'smokeless' industry that would produce a large influx of global capital which could be used to fund other sectors of the economy (Freitag 1996).

## The global imaginary of tourism poles

Typically, Dominican tourism poles consist of physically isolated conglomerates of all-inclusive gated resorts to which most Dominicans have highly restricted access, and to which locals are admitted almost exclusively as service workers. The stark distinction between life inside the resort areas and in the surrounding communities is a distinctive feature of these touristic borderlands. As some tourism and globalization theorists have described, the economic and social processes that characterize these spaces function to create distinct global sites, sub-national spaces that can bypass the nation socially, economically, politically, and ideologically (Harvey 1990; Sassen 1998). Alternate rules and codes of behaviour, in addition to the highly constructed 'natural' landscapes, can create a dramatic rupture from the local or national context as one moves between them.

The ways these tourism poles can create distinct global borderlands in the imaginary of Dominicans is humorously expressed in a recent, and highly popular, Dominican movie by Director José Pintor entitled 'Sanky Panky', a local term used to describe men who move to tourist beach areas in an attempt to advance socially and economically by developing romantic relationships with wealthy foreign women (Pintor 2008). The main character, Genaro, played by popular Dominican comedic actor Fausto Mata, is frustrated with the highly limited economic opportunities in his small home community, and decides to follow the example of a childhood friend and become a wealthy man through marriage with an older foreign woman.

Through his journey to La Romana, a primary tourism pole on the south coast, Genaro implements his scheme of social advancement by securing a job in an exclusive beach resort, a position which affords him the opportunity to meet and begin courting a visiting blonde *gringa* from New York (according to his friends, the 'best kind' of *gringa*). While his journey involves much hilarity, including many tragic–comic situations in which the protagonist suffers endless abuses and injustices at the hands of the bumbling tourists, the epic movie resonates with many Dominicans in its depiction of Genaro's economic frustrations, his vivid dreams of international migration, and his decision to move to a coastal tourism area as a last-ditch strategy to find a better life.

Many elements of this narrative are reflected in the lives of people who migrate to tourism areas throughout the Dominican Republic. One key element is the belief that tourism areas are social contexts in which global norms, interests, and rules govern the social interactions occurring within them. In essence,

crossing into these global borderlands, as Genaro does, while certainly treacherous, enables different opportunities and alternative realities that are more
closely connected to the world beyond the island. Indeed, in the interviews we
conducted with Dominican male sex workers, this alternative spatial reality of
tourism areas was evident in a number of ways. The following exchange, which
occurred between a Dominican male sex worker and a researcher for our study,
serves as a provocative example of this narrative construction of tourism areas as
global cultural spaces:

INTERVIEWER:  Have you ever lived in another country?
PARTICIPANT:  Only in La Romana. [Laughs]
INTERVIEWER:  [Laughs] Well, La Romana is a different country. Don't doubt it.

It is the shared understanding behind this man's configuration of the tourism
area of La Romana as a foreign country that makes his joke funny, since while
he clearly understands that his travel to La Romana is not a true instance of
international travel, it symbolically partakes in these qualities, since La Romana
is *like* 'a different country'. In his humorous rendition, which is immediately
reciprocated by the interviewer (also Dominican), migration to La Romana
symbolically *stands in for* global movement, even as such movement is clearly not
achieved in reality. Importantly, the global imaginary that permeates tourist
spaces occurs not only because of the distinct cultural and social features of
these areas, nor is it a mere function of the fact that international tourists are
present in large numbers in these spaces. These areas are global because they
are imagined jumping off points for Dominican dreams of global mobility;
they are spaces of hoped-for transitions to a different reality that, however
mythological, holds strong cultural sway for Dominicans. Thus, touristic borderlands are not only magnets for Dominican labour migrants in search of
informal sector opportunities, they are also spaces of fantasy production that
permit experimentation and vicarious engagement with global social and sexual
mores.

This magnetic characteristic of tourism areas is evident demographically. In
our study, we surveyed 199 male sex workers, of whom 191 were residing in
either Santo Domingo or Boca Chica at the time of the interview. Of these, 98
(51 per cent) were originally from other, mostly rural, parts of the country. The
internal migrations of the Santo Domingo and Boca Chica residents who originated elsewhere are shown in Figure 7.1. Forty per cent of the sex workers who
were residing in Santo Domingo at the time of the interview originated from
other parts of the country, whereas 73 per cent of Boca Chica residents originated
elsewhere.

While these demographic trends show patterns in population movement, they
tell us little of the experience of these internal migrants. We therefore turn to the
in-depth interviews with labour migrants to understand the meaning of movements
within and between touristic borderlands.

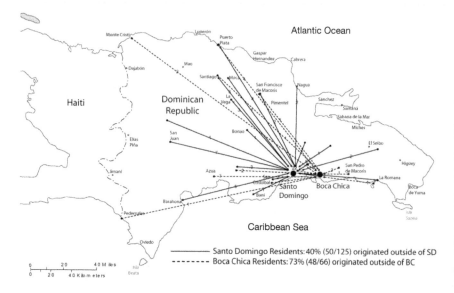

*Figure 7.1* Internal migratory pathways of Dominican male sex workers (n=98)

## Migration to and from the tourism poles

Like Genaro in the aforementioned film, most migrant families, runaway or homeless youth, and single young men and women move towards the *polos turísticos* seeking economic stability. The all-inclusive nature of the resorts creates some formal wage jobs for local service providers (such as maids or entertainment staff), but foreigners occupy most of the skilled positions, and the majority of migrants work in menial or seasonal jobs in the informal economy of the beach around these *polos*. Unlike Genaro, who purposely migrated to become a 'Sanky Panky', many migrant children and youth are readily socialized and incorporated into income-generating activities normatively declared to be a 'crime' – a process Castells (1998: 71) has aptly called the 'perverse integration' resulting from global economic processes. That is, when global economic processes severely constrain the opportunity structures of poor people producing behavioural outcomes that are stigmatized or non-normative, certain behaviours might be redefined as crimes to which individuals – rather than global systems – should be accountable.

As several anthropological studies of Caribbean sex work have demonstrated (Farmer 1992; Kane 1993; Kempadoo 1999; Kreniske 1997; Padilla 2007b), one of the by-products of the increasing mobility of the rural poor is that young migrants to urban and tourism areas are often left without a supportive safety net and with few employment options. Under these conditions, some may come to view the pervasive opportunities for transactional sex with foreigners as the 'easiest' way of making ends meet. Many of these individuals also suffer at the hands of the local authorities and *Policía Turística* (Tourism Police), who tend to view them as 'delinquents' and a potential source of danger to the tourists, rather than as the human resources upon which the entire industry depends.

In our ethnographic research, even when entire families migrated, children and young men were often expected by their parents to contribute money to the household through work, and consequently many of them described the need to *buscársela* ('to look for it', meaning to make ends meet) through informal jobs on the beach. Although these individuals are not considered street children per se, they often described spending most of their days on the beach looking for a range of economic opportunities, and some experienced their first sex-for-money exchanges in this way. Some sex workers told stories of moving from the *campo* (countryside) alone, some of them fleeing violence and abuse at home, becoming *niños de la calle* (street kids), and finding intermittent informal sector jobs as *limpiabotas* (shoe-shiners) or *chiriperos* (street vendors). Often these runaways followed a migratory path that took them to the beach or urban tourism areas, where they could establish contacts with tourists. Rodrigo, a sex worker interviewed in the tourist town of Boca Chica, told a story that is illustrative of many of these themes.

When Rodrigo was seven years old, his parents separated. From then on, he was constantly moving between different homes – his grandmother's, his mother's, and his father's. By age 12, the death of his mother increased his housing and emotional instability and he contemplated suicide. He was finally kicked out by his overtly strict and physically and verbally abusive father and moved to the beach at age 14.

> I was 14 [when I arrived in Boca Chica, a tourist town]. I ate a lot of fish heads left on the plates [by tourists], slept in the lawn chairs, was hungry often, had bad times, rough times. And I overcame those, did some bad things like stealing, living with men, living with women, a lot of things that were not pleasant and don't want to remember it either.

Rodrigo's involvement in sexual encounters at an early age is not uncommon among runaway children in touristic borderlands. Unlike those sex workers who migrated as adults seeking economic opportunities, including those provided by sex work, runaway children lack family support systems and are socialized earlier into the sex economy of tourism areas out of economic desperation, either at the suggestion of more experienced peers or due to an unsolicited offer from a potential client. The growth of the tourism industry has only intensified this intersection of internal migration and sex work. Furthermore, as young migrants are increasingly likely to seek or find the opportunity to engage in relatively lucrative sexual exchanges with foreigners, many of them begin to entertain the fantasy of continuing the migratory path out of the country.

## Being 'taken away'

Many sex workers in our project spoke of steady clients who hired them for several days or upon consecutive visits to the Dominican Republic. Furthermore, sex workers often discussed the advantages of developing relationships that could result in future cash remittances from abroad. More information on these encounters can be found elsewhere (Padilla 2007b). Here we are interested in the discursive integration of migration desires and sex work, since making a tourist fall in love frequently becomes a strategy – however improbable – for leaving the country.

In responding to the question of how he defines himself, Carlos, 23 years old, who grew up poor in the countryside and migrated to the beach at age 20, vividly expressed the desire to leave the country as a fundamental part of his identity:

> I define myself as someone that is looking for a future, you understand? But I unfortunately don't want to live here. Because here you are waiter. You can't—if I'm going on vacation—you can't even go to Haiti. You can't, with the small salary of a waiter. You will not be able to buy a car. But there [abroad] it's different. So, I believe I'm one that is trying to find a woman, or something, to fall in love with me and take me abroad ... So I define myself as—as 'I'm Carlos and I want to get out of the country'.

The hope of leaving the country through a relationship with an international tourist has been documented in other studies of Dominican sex workers (De Moya *et al.* 1992; De Moya and Garcia 1996, 1998; Cabezas 1999; Brennan 2004). Similarly, in this study, as with Carlos, many male sex workers expressed their desire to leave the country and the hope that someone would fall in love with them and 'take me away' (*llevarme*). Since only in few cases did male workers consider the possibility of falling in love with another man, their romantic interests and migration hopes were almost exclusively centred on female tourists.

Consequently, an important part of their sex work was getting the client emotionally invested in the encounter, since besides increasing the economic benefits beyond a single sexual encounter, this opened the imagined possibility, albeit remote, of international immigration. Given their self-identification as heterosexual men, participants often spoke of an older *gringa* that would fall in love and discussed scripts or performances that had worked for them. Mario, who had done sex work at the beach for the last three years, discussed his approach:

> In my life, a day for me, I get up around nine, come here to the beach, look at the women, whatever, find one. Well, I invite her to the disco and something, go out, we go Dutch. Well if I teach her to dance, given that she is a tourist or something, and she likes me, and when you realize it, we've

spent the night ... They fall in love with you easily. It's more likely – a 60 per cent chance – that she'll be enchanted by you and stay with you. If they are going to stay two or three weeks, they are always with you.

Successful or not, the romantic relationship is from the beginning geographically bounded and structured by the social, cultural and economic differences between tourists and sex workers. Unable to travel abroad, long-term relations are dependent on the client's willingness to visit the country or desire to pursue the relationship. According to our participants, tourists did, in fact, fall in love on occasion and promise to send the immigration paperwork necessary, but more often than not they did not follow up with this or return to the country. There was a consciousness among sex workers that the spatial and social separation after the love affair could end with the tourist 'forgetting' the sex worker after returning home. Almost as if it were a part of the encounter's social script, one sex worker commented, 'They [the tourists] offer you a trip, *even if they don't carry it out*'. Indeed, it may be that the fantasy of the offer is a part of what is being purchased by the tourist – akin to what sociologist Elizabeth Bernstein (2007a, 2007b) has described as 'bounded authenticity'. The spatial and temporal boundaries that surround the encounter allow the tourist to entertain a romantic fantasy that functions to fulfil desires that are eroticized precisely because of their bounded, finite nature.

Sex workers are aware of the bounded nature of tourist fantasies. Even though Mario wanted women to fall in love with him, his plan of finding a wealthy tourist to take him away was tempered by his consciousness of the transient nature of tourism relationships, and the fact that when the romance eventually faded, his financial need would remain. He also was aware that the fantasy of the 'wealthy' client who could radically transform one's material condition was a myth:

> There are many people who think that all tourists that come here have a lot of money, and that is a lie. 40 per cent. ... 60 per cent of tourists that come here, let's say to Boca Chica, anywhere, and who work six months, a year, to come here, don't come with much money, and sometimes, the person is here and you meet her, you like her and she likes you, sometimes she's pretty, and you are with her. But even if she's pretty, then, the first days you are going to feel good, but then after it's been two weeks or more, and you know she is a foreigner and she came on vacation, and you know she's with you and she's not paying you, even if she's Princess Diana, you know you are going to feel dissatisfied, dissatisfied.

For some sex workers, this consciousness of the transient nature of tourism translated into the awareness and development of alternative sources of income. Juan, 17 years old, married and with a child, felt proud of his work in construction as a plaster specialist. He had engaged in sex work for the last two years as a way of increasing his income, especially when construction work was slow. He expressed a deep desire to travel abroad. When asked about what he was doing to make it possible, he responded: 'I make tourists fall in love, the *gringas*'. Nevertheless, Juan was also aware of the limitations of his reliance on sex work with tourists and the need to create alternative sources of income, since sex work was a dead-end road:

> Being a *bugarrón* or sanky panky [local terms for sex workers] is a fantasy because it's never going to lead to anything. And if there are not tourists or anything, what are they going to aspire to? When the tourists from abroad don't come, what are they going to do? Be stuck. One has to think always in the future; one needs to have something, you know. I thank God that he gave me my brain and I already have a profession.

Paradoxically, as described in the next section, while being 'stuck' in the fantasy of a better life through tourists was generally regarded with scepticism, the motivation to engage tourists at a more intimate level also made some sex workers more marketable in the tourism sector by increasing their interpersonal skills and even their options for upward mobility.

## 'Opening up' to the global

Although tourism has created a variety of jobs in the service area at hotels, the beach itself constitutes the most important subsistence site for the large majority of residents in towns close to the resorts. As an interviewee put it, 'It is rare that someone from here, Boca Chica, doesn't live off the beach'. Nonetheless, the transformation of former fishing towns into global tourism poles has resulted in the development of a service sector with particular skills and worldviews. Many respondents talked at length about how the social interactions with tourism had changed, both positively and negatively, their ideas, behaviours, and abilities. Some described their experiences in terms of 'mind opening', 'economic improvement', or 'gaining knowledge about other cultures'. This is illustrated by Martín, 23 years old:

> Here in Boca Chica one opens up a lot ... Any person that works here *opens up* because that person has to ... Sometimes a situation makes one do things, not so much for money, but tourism makes many things outside of the normal.

'Opening up' was facilitated by the fact that the Dominican tourism sector has become increasingly diversified, and now attracts tourists from a very wide range of countries of origin. Most participants had strong opinions about clients of different cultures, nationalities, and races, but the close interactions with tourists from many countries gave these men a cosmopolitan attitude. In a country where bilingualism is almost exclusively a characteristic of the upper classes or 'Dominicanyorks', informants often boasted about their ability to communicate in multiple languages. Based on fieldwork experience, many of them were, indeed, able to sustain simple conversations focused on the tourist's basic needs, such as food, shopping, hotels, or recreation. They also boasted the ability to recognize cultural traits and particularities such as facial features, clothing, eating habits, or demeanour, which were regarded as skills to better target tourists. Indeed, the ability to detect such distinctions can have a direct effect on income, if one is skilled at developing rapport by picking up on regional or linguistic cues.

As participants explained, language skills and knowledge of the global are also useful for dealing with the fickle dimensions of the tourism industry and the decrease in sex work opportunities during low tourism season. Despite frequently repeating stories about clients who gave them fabulous sums of money in exchange for sexual encounters, most respondents did not depend exclusively on sex work. Their income usually came from sex work in combination with a range of other jobs in the informal economy, for example, selling crafts, renting chairs, providing tours, or waiting tables. But the skills gained in 'emotion work' with tourists were relatively portable, that is, they improved productive possibilities for income generation in a range of services, thereby providing a defence against the inherent uncertainties of the Dominican pleasure-based economy.

In summary, opening up to the global in these borderlands provided young male sex workers with skills for expanding their income opportunities and for experiencing social encounters with global travellers and their cultures, and cultivated portable qualities that they could use instrumentally in other productive activities. However, as demonstrated in the following section, these experiences were not without perceived social or moral costs, since these men were constrained by local geography, 'stuck' within the borderlands. This meant that their experiences of global realities were always vicarious, transient, and tempered by their moral ties to local definitions of normalcy.

### The price of 'easy money'

Tourism makes the beach both a site for opening up to global cultures and a site for contesting more conservative social norms of masculinity, femininity, and sexuality. In this contested process, participants expressed concern over the negative influences of 'easy money' on youth. As Orlando, 21 years old, stated, one's productive involvement in tourism exposed workers such as himself, whether they liked it or not, to the negative underbelly of the industry:

As they say, one doesn't study what one wants, just what one can. I mean, economically, you know? A person is in this environment, in tourism, you know, which is the principle base of this, and from tourism comes the corruption, prostitution, drug addiction, everything. So it's hard.

Similarly, Gabriel, 32 years old, who was married with three children, began exchanging sex for money soon after he ran away from home at age 11. He felt strongly about the influence of tourism on young men, who could get young men *acostumbrado* (used to) a world of easy money without being aware of the social and moral consequences of doing so:

> The tourist gets a boy used to it. How? Because if I'm a person, let's say, and I'm getting 200 or 300 pesos daily [approximately $11 to $17 US dollars in 2001], and you come and tell me, 'Come with me and I'm going to give you 4,000 or 5,000 pesos [$235 to $294 US dollars]', and you're giving 4,000 or 5,000 pesos to that boy, that boy is going to get used to a life. What life? To drinking every day, he gets used to drugs, he gets used to this and gets used to that, you hear? And from there comes the problem: when that boy doesn't have a dime [*un chele*], he robs the tourist.

For some participants, the beach also constituted a site of danger for the reputation of young men and women. Raul, 51 years old, had worked on the beach since his family moved from the country side to Boca Chica at age 11. He had been a sex worker for nearly 40 years, but at the time of interview, he only worked finding sex workers for tourists in exchange for a small fee (approximately US$7). Although he observed that sex work on the beach had been going on for a long time, he felt the situation was deteriorating rapidly:

> Okay, I'm going to explain it to you. There's so much corruption here in Boca Chica, in addition to the little respect that parents have for their kids ... Let's say, I have my three boys and a girl, here nobody will see my children here on the beach *buscándosela* [looking for it, meaning engaging in sex work] and *sinvergüenzerías* [doing shameful things], you see? Because the first thing I say, you see, is 'I don't want to see you on the beach. Now, when you want to go to the beach, I'll take you.'

Respondents often linked changes in the social organization of sex work, gender relations, and sexual norms to changes in tourism. According to one participant, for example, the presence of international tourism to the Dominican Republic altered the nature of sexual encounters in the Dominican Republic.

PARTICIPANT: [Sexual relations] are different because, I say, the Americans came here with that, with that fever here and they paid, in those days they gave gifts, so they implanted that. *Ellos fueron los que hicieron los trabajadores sexuales.* (*They were the ones that made the sex workers*).
INTERVIEWER: You say that the tourist is the one who has influenced ... ?
PARTICIPANT: Yes, yes, the tourist has come here, and the people said 'Okay, over there it is the place where the Americans, where—They buy you

clothes, they bring you tennis shoes, they pay you dollars ... So, then, let's do it. What is it that you have to do?'

In other instances, men claimed that an increase in openly gay tourism had transformed sex work and the social interactions between gay men and sex workers. For example, one man argued that these changes had resulted in a decrease in sex work on the beach and an increase in male strippers at dance clubs. These statements reflected an awareness of changing sexual geographies as a result of the sex tourism industry, which was often expressed in conjunction with anxieties over the impact of tourism on the social and sexual life of either themselves or Dominican youth more generally.

In sum, entry into touristic borderlands was viewed by these men as a somewhat treacherous transformative activity. Like liminal experiences themselves, these areas were spaces for play and transgression, but while this flexibility allowed men to learn about alternative global realities, they raised questions about the lasting influences of such experiences on personhood, behaviour, and moral integrity. Easy money was therefore a deceptive phenomenon, providing young men a safety valve for material needs in a difficult work environment, while getting them used to the seductive dangers of tourism environments. For the tourist, these dangers were often transient escapist experiences; for Dominicans tied irrevocably to the local, they were a permanent reality that raised moral questions and dilemmas.

## HIV and AIDS

In addition to disruptions in the social organization of gender and sexuality, studies in a variety of international settings have shown that male labour migration and international sex tourism increase HIV risk, as measured by both frequencies of sexual risk behaviours and HIV infection rates. In the Caribbean, some epidemiological evidence suggests an ecological connection between tourism and HIV/AIDS, since regions with the greatest tourism development tend to show the greatest impact from the epidemic (Camara 2001). Nonetheless, the lack of comprehensive epidemiological, behavioural, and ethnographic data on HIV transmission and the social context of risk behaviour makes the task of determining the impact of tourism on the AIDS epidemic a difficult task at best. Although many studies have examined HIV risks among sex workers in tourism areas, the diversification of modalities of sex work and the pervasive cultural logic of sexual-economic exchanges in tourism areas creates barriers to understanding the nuances of sexual risk in different kinds of exchanges or sex work environments. In fact, some of the participants in this study believed that prostitution was linked to HIV in particular kinds of environments. For example, in response to a question about the presence of AIDS in Boca Chica, one sex worker argued:

Yes, [there is] a lot of disease. But there is not much AIDS here in Boca Chica. The women around here are very careful with the gringos. But there are a good number of women that hustle in the bars, only with Dominicans, for 50 or 75 pesos. They are in fact the ones sick. They don't care about anything. But I don't go to those places.

In addition to categorizing female sex workers as high or low depending on their workspace and nationality of their clients, male sex workers in this study also assessed the 'riskiness' of their partners based on their presumed exposure to global sex tourism. Thus, while the HIV risk was considered high among *mujeres de la playa* (women of the beach), it was thought to be low among *mujeres de la casa* (stay-home women). This produced a selective approach to condom use that was influenced by both women's presumed 'exposure' to the tourism industry, as well as to the spatial location of the transaction. As an example of this, one participant explained his different patterns of condom use in different social geographies: 'I have had sexual relations without condoms. Not with women here *at the beach* but with women *de por mi casa* (from my neighbourhood)'. The juxtaposition of 'at the beach' with 'my neighbourhood' reveal an implicit mapping of HIV risk within different social terrains, and the ways that people attempt to avoid the contagion of tourism – in terms of both its moral and disease-based risks – by managing their social and sexual distance from high-tourism areas.

These observations strongly suggest that future research on tourism and HIV/AIDS in the Caribbean should explore the spatial, social and economic contexts of tourism areas as a means to describe how space is subjectively mapped onto subjective models of sexual risk or 'danger', and how these differences influence sexual practices and decisions, such as the selection of sexual partners. Furthermore, future research needs to understand tourism areas not as pathological environments, but as spaces of perceived possibility which promote new kinds of erotic and sexual experiences with a variety of consequences for specific individuals. For example, some participants in this study reported learning about condom use through sexual interactions with tourists who introduced the condom or insisted on condom use. Carlos, a 37 year old who had engaged in sex work since he was in his early 20s, observed that,

> I learned [to use condoms] because the women I first hung out with were tourists and they demanded condoms. They were teaching me how to put it on and as the world is more complicated with diseases, I have tried to have condoms in the bike [hold] or my room always.

Given that few studies have been conducted among tourists who pay for sex work, it is unclear whether tourists arriving from countries with higher rates of HIV prevention knowledge and condom use might provide the basis for the diffusion of HIV protective strategies among local populations. Indeed, the lack of HIV prevention campaigns for local male sex workers suggests that ad hoc interactions with foreign clients may be a significant influence on the 'safety' or 'risk' of local tourism workers.

## Conclusion

The spatial and social qualities of touristic borderlands have only begun to be explored in the social scientific literature. While tourism theorists have long described the performance of the local for visiting foreign guests (MacCannell 1976; Crick 1989; Urry 1995, 2002), they have less often examined the local cultural reverberations of global tourism spaces or migrant experiences within and between these particularly constructed social environments. Our ethnographic reflections in this chapter, drawing on research with Dominican male sex workers, suggest that these spaces are experienced by locals ambivalently: as multidimensional spaces of global possibilities, cosmopolitan attitudes, and opportunities for productive activity, on the one hand, and as zones of moral and physical danger, on the other. Through the narratives of participants, we also discern the felt tension between fantasies of global mobility on the part of locals and the undeniable fact that they are 'stuck' – a tension which structures much of the social interaction that occurs within the borderlands. While intimate strategies of love and romance are used by young men as means to leverage the remote possibility of being taken away – and, indeed, may promote useful skills for professional advancement within the service sector – their keen awareness of the situational, transient, bounded quality of these romantic connections led some young men to seek more immediate strategies for material advancement.

Future ethnographic research on touristic borderlands should aim to understand how passage through these spaces is transforming social relations, sexuality, and engagements with the global. Furthermore, while HIV research globally has shown consistent associations between migration and viral transmission, relatively little ethnographic work has been conducted to understand how migratory environments are understood or experienced as social spaces, a fact which reduces the relevance of much research for the design of meaningful programs or interventions. Much of the existing research also neglects a consideration of tourism areas as particular kinds of destinations for local or national labour migration, with potentially significant implications for HIV transmission. We believe the first step in such research should be close engagement with the narratives of labour migrants to tourism areas, and the development of ethnographically grounded theories of the social structure of touristic borderlands.

## References

Benoît, C. (1999) 'Sex, AIDS, migration, and prostitution: human trafficking in the Caribbean', *New West Indian Guide*, 73(342.

Bernstein, E. (2007a) 'Buying and selling the "Girlfriend Experience": the social and subjective contours of market intimacy', in M. B. Padilla, J. S. Hirsch, M. Munoz-Laboy, R. E. Sember and R. G. Parker (eds), *Love and Globalization: Transformations of Intimacy in the Contemporary World*, Nashville: Vanderbilt University Press.

——(2007b) *Temporarily Yours: Intimacy, Authenticity, and the Commerce of Sex*, Chicago: University of Chicago Press.

Brennan, D. (2004) *What's Love Got to Do with It? Transnational Desires and Sex Tourism in the Dominican Republic*, Durham and London: Duke University Press.

Bronfman, M., Camposortega, S. and Medina, H. (1989) *Myths and Realities of the Migration-AIDS Relationship: the Case of Mexican Migration to the United States*. Paper presented at the International Conference on AIDS, Mexico City, Mexico.

Broring, G. and Van Duifhuizen, R. (1993) 'Mobility and the spread of HIV/AIDS: a challenge to health promotion', *AIDS Health Promotion Exchange*, 1, 1–3.

Cabezas, A. L. (1999) 'Women's work is never done: sex tourism in Sosúa, the Dominican Republic', in K. Kempadoo (ed.), *Sun, Sex, and Gold: Tourism and Sex Work in the Caribbean*, Boulder: Rowman & Littlefield.

Camara, B. (2001) *20 Years of the HIV/AIDS Epidemic in the Caribbean*, Port of Spain: CAREC-SPSTI.

Castells, M. (1998) *End of Millennium*, Malden: Blackwell.

Crick, M. (1989) 'Representations of international tourism in the social sciences: sun, sex, sights, savings, and servility', *Annual Review of Anthropology*, 18, 307–44.

De Moya, A. and Garcia, R. (1998) 'Three decades of male sex work in Santo Domingo', in P. Aggleton (ed.), *Men Who Sell Sex: International Perspectives on Male Prostitution and AIDS*, London: Taylor & Francis.

De Moya, E. A. and Garcia, R. (1996) 'AIDS and the enigma of bisexuality in the Dominican Republic', in P. Aggleton (ed.), *Bisexualities and AIDS: International Perspectives*, Bristol, Pennsylvania: Taylor & Francis.

De Moya, E. A., Garcia, R., Fadul, R. and Herold, E. (1992) *Report: Sosua Sanky-Pankies and Female Sex Workers: An Exploratory Study*, Santo Domingo: La Universidad Autonoma de Santo Domingo.

Decosas, J. (1998) 'Labour migration and HIV epidemics in Africa', *AIDS Analysis Africa*, 8 (5), 6–7.

Farmer, P. (1992) *AIDS and Accusation: Haiti and the Geography of Blame*, 1st edn, Berkeley: University of California Press.

Freitag, T. G. (1996) 'Tourism and the transformation of a Dominican coastal community', *Urban Anthropology and Studies of Cultural Systems and World Economic Development*, 25, 225–58.

Georges, E. (1990) *The Making of a Transnational Community: Migration, Development, and Cultural Change in the Dominican Republic*, New York: Columbia University Press.

Grasmuck, S. and Pessar, P. (1991) *Between Two Islands: Dominican International Migration*, Berkeley: University of California Press.

Harvey, D. (1990) *The Condition of Postmodernity*, Cambridge: Blackwell.

Jochelson, K., Mothibeli, M. and Leger, J. P. (1991) 'Human Immunodeficiency Virus and migrant labor in South Africa', *International Journal of Health Services*, 21(1), 157–73.

Kane, S. C. (1993) 'Prostitution and the military: planning AIDS intervention in Belize', *Social Science & Medicine*, 36(7), 965–79.

Kempadoo, K. (ed.) (1999) *Sun, Sex and Gold: Tourism and Sex Work in the Caribbean*, New York: Rowman & Littlefield.

Kreniske, J. (1997) 'AIDS in the Dominican Republic: anthropological reflections on the social nature of disease', in G. C. Bond, J. Kreniske, I. Susser and J. Vincent (eds), *AIDS in Africa and the Caribbean*, Boulder: Westview.

Lozano, W. (1997) 'Dominican Republic: informal economy, the State, and the urban poor', in A. Portes, C. Dore and P. Landolt (eds), *The Urban Caribbean: Transition to the New Global Economy*, Baltimore: Johns Hopkins University Press.

MacCannell, D. (1976) *The Tourist: A New Theory of the Leisure Class*, New York: Shocken Books.

Morel, E. and Mejía, M. (1996) 'Los impactos de los desalojos: la constitución o reconstitución de las identidades', in A. Navarro García (ed.), *Antología Urbana de Ciudad Alternativa*, Santo Domingo: Ciudad Alternativa.

Oficina Nacional de Estadística (2004) Resultados Generales, Santo Domingo, D.N. Resultados Definitivos. *VIII Censo Nacional de Población y Vivienda 2002*. Online. Available from: www.one.gob.do (accessed 16 March 16, 2007).

Padilla, M. B. (2007a) *Caribbean Pleasure Industry: Tourism, Sexuality, and AIDS in the Dominican Republic*, Chicago and London: University of Chicago Press.

Padilla, M. B. (2007b) '"Western Union daddies" and their quest for authenticity: an ethnographic study of the Dominican gay sex tourism industry', *Journal of Homosexuality*, 53(1–2), 241–75.

Pintor, J. (2008) *Sanky Panky*, Dominican Republic.

Sassen, S. (1998) *Globalization and its Discontents. Essays on the New Mobility of People and Money*, New York: New Press.

Urry, J. (1995) *Consuming Places*, New York: Routledge.

—— (2002) *The Tourist Gaze*, London: Sage.

World Bank Development Data Group (DECDG) (2006) Dominican Republic at-a-Glance [Electronic Version]. *Development Economics*. Online. Available from: devdata.worldbank.org/AAG/dom_aag.pdf (accessed 16 March 2007).

# Chapter 8

# Rice, rams and remittances

*Bumsters* and female tourists in The Gambia

*Stella Nyanzi and Ousman Bah*

The Gambia has a reputation as a tourist destination where beach boys offer sexual services to female tourists, often in the hope of establishing partnerships which provide opportunities for migration to the West (Brown 1992; Ebron 2002; Nyanzi *et al.* 2005; Fleming 2006). Criticising traditional tourism studies which limit their focus to male tourists who 'sexually exploit' female sex workers (Oppermann 1999; Ryan 1999), it is increasingly recognised that sexual inter-action and exchange also takes place between male local providers and women tourists (cf. Brown 1992; Phillips 1999; Kempadoo 2001; Ebron 2002; Jeffreys 2003; Nyanzi *et al.* 2005; Taylor 2006; Bauer 2007; Jennaway 2008).

A feminist analytical framework posited by McCormick (1994) categorises stu-dies of these relationships as either radical – because local players are situated as exploited victims of powerful Western nations, or liberal – because the relationships are interpreted as sites of sexual empowerment, pleasure, experience and fulfil-ment. While this dichotomy is useful as a heuristic device that allows explanation of complex processes, it is also too simplistic to capture the inherent contradictions, flux, ambivalences and dynamic character of these sexual interactions.

Rather than start with the premise of exploitation, this chapter explores rea-sons given by, and experiences of, *bumsters* (Gambian beach boys) entering into sexual liaisons with female tourists. Understanding *bumsters'* emic perspective is a crucial precursor to analysing what Western women encounter when they fall for locals while on holiday and the sexual risks that both sides are prepared to take.

## Mobility, tourism and HIV/AIDS in The Gambia

With a population of 1.7 million, The Gambia is the smallest country in West Africa. Rural–urban migration has facilitated rapid urbanisation, particularly in the coastal urban-peripherals of Greater Banjul Area, and Kombos St. Mary's. Regular cyclical migration is patterned along two seasons which revolve around the agricultural cycle and the tourism boom season between November and April. Responding to developments in the tourism industry, young men season-ally travel to urban coastal areas to tap into the tourist trade by offering various entrepreneurial services.

Tourism is a major sector of The Gambia's economy, supporting over 10,000 direct and indirect jobs and earning US$39 million in foreign exchange (Department of State for Finance and Economic Affairs 2006). Currently, 87 per cent of annual arrivals are from the UK, the Netherlands, Spain and Scandinavia. Although there are plans to promote The Gambia as a destination for cultural, heritage, health and eco-tourism most current investors are international tour companies specialising in short-term holiday package tours (Ashley *et al.* 2000; Ebron 2002).

The first case of HIV in The Gambia was acknowledged in 1986. However, the initial national response was dominated by silence and denial in a bid to protect the tourist industry. There is widespread doubt about the incurability of AIDS,[1] and denial of HIV infection as a Gambian reality (Shaw and Jawo 2000). According to UNAIDS (2007), HIV prevalence among adults aged 15–49 years is 2.4 per cent and transmission is mainly through heterosexual sex. Among women attending antenatal clinics, prevalence of HIV-1 is 1.0 per cent, and HIV-2 is 0.8 per cent (Van der Loeff *et al.* 2003).

## The study methods

Ethics clearance for the present study was provided by the London School of Hygiene and Tropical Medicine, and local approval was secured via the Gambian National Council for Arts and Culture. Data collection triangulated participant observation, 45 repeat interviews, 12 focus group discussions, media content analysis, and review of policy rhetoric and text.[2] During repeat interviews, we compiled sexual histories of 20 *bumsters* operating in the Senegambia tourist region, on BB and Kotu beaches. We observed their interactions with diverse groups including tourists, tour operators, airport and hotel employees, policemen, family and other *bumsters*. Because the fieldwork extended over a considerable period, we were able to initiate contact, forge relationships, build rapport and establish trust with different individuals, allowing us to map trajectories of social, economic and sexual interactions forged between *bumsters* and tourists.[3]

During initial participant observation around Senegambia area, purposive sampling of *bumsters* fitting stereotypical images portrayed in local media provided the initial study sample. We approached individuals[4] to participate in a series of repeat interviews. During these sessions, we asked participants to introduce us to relevant others whose experiences would confirm, contradict or add new dimensions to emerging narratives of *bumster* sexualities.

### Locating 'the bumster as a problem' construct in policy and society

A critical review of key national policy documents revealed that *bumsters* are constructed as a problematic social category in official discourse. In the 'Strategic Tourism Master Plan', they are, for example, described as 'the *bumster* problem' and viewed as a sign of irresponsible tourism (Gambia Tourism Authority 2005:9). The *Poverty Reduction Strategy Paper: 2008–2011* categorises them as a negative social issue – 'the *bumster* problem', and lists them among the weaknesses and constraints facing the tourism industry (Department of State for Finance and Economic Affairs 2006:65).

*Bumsters* are targets of intensive campaigns to reduce and eventually eliminate their perceived negative activities within tourism (cf. Nyanzi *et al.* 2005). While the Gambian Tourism Authority issued a series of public initiatives aimed at highlighting the negative impacts of these beach boys on the tourism industry, Western tourism companies and travel media have colluded in portraying images of *bumsters* 'construed around the notions of mistrust, deceit … and disingenuousness' (Lawson and Jaworski 2007:79). In society more generally, there are diverse reactions towards the activities of *bumsters* ranging from disapproval, to ambivalence, to support (Ebron 2002; Jassey 2005; Nyanzi *et al.* 2005), depending on whether individuals stand to gain from the profits through diffusion or trickle-down effects.

### Who is a bumster? Transcending stereotypes

*Bumster* is, however, an ambiguous and ambivalent label. In order not to be derogatory, alienate potential participants, or align our study with oppressive structures, we aimed at an operational definition which was value-free and emically correct. Thus, *bumster*, at the simplest level of meaning referred to young men who strategically position themselves in areas visited by tourists in order to initiate interaction.

Analysis of policy documents revealed underlying assumptions in conceptualisations of policymakers, stakeholders in the tourist industry and youth organisation workers that were not necessarily reflected in the lived realities of many *bumsters* in our study. These included assumptions that *bumsters* were unemployed, uneducated, from poor family backgrounds, irreligious, and forceful in their approach to tourists. Furthermore, *bumsters* were often presented as petty criminals who operated haphazardly, with neither plan nor strategy. The profiles, life histories, experiences and narratives of our study participants challenge these assumptions as unfounded within the reality of *bumsters*.

Sending-communities of the study participants were diverse (see Figure 8.1). While 23 *bumsters* resided in coastal beach environs, a few others travelled from areas further inland. During the tourist season, all were urban-based. Many lived as visitors or dependants of relatives and friends with compounds in the Kombos coastal area. A few (9/45) belonged to families with property in the tourist area. The majority (26/45) were either urban migrants or seasonal immigrants who originated from rural provinces. Four participants operating on one beach were refugees from Liberia and Sierra Leone. On the extreme end were *bumsters* who were returnees from abroad. Deportees were legally forced back, often from Germany, Sweden, or the UK because of immigration violations, crime or

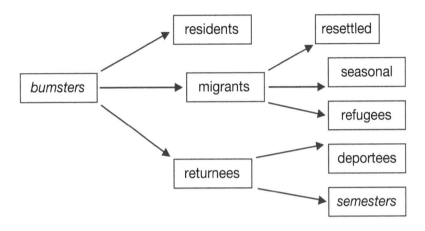

*Figure 8.1* Spatial typology of *bumsters*

marital discord. *Semesters* often chose to return either on holiday, at the end of their visa, or expiration of resident permits. Unable to independently raise resources, they resumed *bumsing* with the hope of making new connections with a Westerner able to transport them abroad again.

A distinct lower cadre of *bumsters* comprised new arrivals on the beach scene who migrated from rural provinces without any urban contacts. Lacking regular accommodation, these individuals must rely on their social skills to penetrate existing networks, and form friendships with residents or other *bumsters*. Those with advanced communication skills can negotiate temporary accommodation usually as non-paying guests, or short-term employees as casual labourers including car-washers, rubbish-pickers, cleaners, brokers, security guards, etc. If such strategies fail, some *bumsters* resort to sleeping in dance halls, at gas-filling stations, on verandas or the beaches. The shanty wooden kiosks on the beach were common hideouts from which homeless *bumsters* emerged early in the mornings. Bathing in the ocean for hygiene purposes left trails of salt residue stuck on their skins, particularly visible under the hot sun. Often hungry and lacking a change of clothes, they quickly lost the potential of attaching themselves to established networks of more seasoned *bumsters*. Participants explained that when outsiders to this subculture referred to dirty, unkempt, or criminal-looking *bumsters*, it was this group under description. Generally, such low-cadre *bumsters* were more upfront about getting money from tourists, and nagged, cajoled, pestered and persisted because their immediate needs were unattended.

While not formally employed, many *bumsters* are involved in the service industry working as unofficial guides, waiters, security, pimps connecting male tourists with local female sex providers, musicians, fishmongers, taxi drivers, craft-sellers, or middlemen assisting tourists purchase items from different markets (Brown 1992; Ebron 2002; Nyanzi *et al.* 2005). *Bumsters* thus juggle casual employment alongside their pursuance of tourists.

Contrary to the notion that *bumsters* are illiterate and uneducated, the majority (32/45) of study participants attained some primary school education, some had 'O' levels, and a few (5/45) had completed high school. All participants had successfully completed Islamic education in *madarassas*. Consistent with the national profile, the majority were Muslims. However many individuals observed the cultural aspects of the religion, without necessarily adhering to the entire doctrinal ethos, moralities and spirituality. *Bumsters* challenged accusations of being uneducated. The ability to speak the English language is a highly desired mark of 'being civilised', higher social class, and a notch up the elitist ladder. Not only did all the *bumsters* in our study speak English, but some even spoke other Western languages including German, French, Dutch and Swedish.

LAMIN: Early school-drop-outs cannot converse for a long time with these tourists.
EBOU: It is not easy to bring a bush-man from the villagers to become an expert at this job. You need some good English – not just speaking what not rubbish, but also understanding if the tourist asks you a question.
OUSBOY: Conversation please. Not only, 'Hello Boss-lady! Can I help you?' [Laughter from others.]
LAMIN: Some boys chant phrases many times in order to remember them, without understanding. But they are the ones who do not go far with tourists.
MALANG: You need school to hassle well.

(Focus group discussion, Kotu Beach, 2006)

Us here, we know it is hard to be in Babylon not knowing the Whiteman's language. It's why we always practise a fine accent which you hear in the films. This is important. But how to do if you have not gone inside in a classroom and sat in front of a blackboard? We have education. Even when it is small, it is there.

(Marena, individual in-depth interview, June 2004)

Education attainment is strongly gendered in The Gambia. Indicators for school enrolment, retention and performance are better for boys than girls at all levels of the education system (Department of State for Education 2004). However education levels are relatively low. The only university in the country opened in 1999.[5] Thus in the emic logic of *bumsters*, their levels of education attainment were not deviant from those of the general Gambian population and they often stressed the structural limitation created by prevailing systemic failures of the post-colonial nation-state to provide widely accessible university education.

Study participants frequently dispelled criticisms of low-education attainment as leading to their vocation as *bumsters*, by variously naming and shaming different public officials holding government positions and yet not going far in school. A common rejoinder was, 'Even our president is a school-drop-out, but he is the most important man in the whole country. No one punishes him for having small-small education'.

Furthermore, it was not uncommon to hear about *bumsters* who successfully interspersed their activities on the beaches with education. A few *bumsed* tourists outside their school schedule – either in the evenings of the tourist season, or during weekends and school vacations. Some older *bumsters* were open about *bumsing* as truants.[6]

The choice to work as a *bumster* is not always perceived as inferior by those who do it. Rather than being the only option available to the most marginal members of society, able-bodied, creative and highly calculating young men make a conscious choice to make a living as *bumsters*. They strategise, improve their technique, and work at perfecting their personal assets in order to succeed at *bumsing*. They invest as individuals and groups in toning their body muscles, grooming their physical presentation, and calculating their outward costume (Phillips 1999; Jassey 2005). The fake white smile, nutty dreads, practised bounce, slow leisurely gait, sexy gaze, sensual cool voice, and rehearsed phrases in fake accents are all strategies to woo over unsuspecting tourist females. Within *bumster* cliques, sharing of tips for enhancing sex appeal while on the job is essential to maintaining membership within networks.

The image of *bumsters* as poor, destitute, suffering youths from struggling families is rife particularly in the international press and electronic media. Possible sources of this false portrayal are the tales of Westerners who fell for the (often exaggerated or even fabricated) plight stories of *bumsters* (Brown 1992; Dahles and Bras 1999; Nyanzi *et al.* 2005). Given that these tales are often unfounded, clichéd, similar across settings, and merely strategies for maximising benefits for individual *bumsters*, it is puzzling that Westerners persist in believing them wholesale.[7]

*Bumsters* go a long way to cultivate storylines of poverty[8]; usually not their own lack but rather that of family and close kin who are presented as solely dependent on this one individual. Usually it is important that the *bumster* is not the object of suffering, but rather presents himself as a responsible, caring, concerned individual upon whose shoulders the family burden solidly sits. And it is too heavy to bear alone, too entrenched to be avoided, thus the urgent desperation for support from a third party. Spinning the stories is well calculated to draw upon the chords of compassion, mercy, and even guilt or shame at attempting to ignore such an immense plight.

It is critical to get the right balance between a well-groomed sexually attractive appearance and the image of belonging to suffering kin; presentable enough to be companionable to wealthy Westerners, whilst still demonstrating 'need' as evidence of requiring financial assistance and support. Jassey (2005) discusses the acquisition of trademark brand name commodities in order to impress tourists, for example, Nike canvas shoes, whilst others have identified a continuum of *bumsters* with sophistication, calculated smoothness, and subtle deception developed over time (Nyanzi *et al.* 2005). Brown (1992) reveals older *bomsas* (an alternative local pronunciation of 'bumster', particularly spoken by people of Mandinka ethnicity) who settle down as entrepreneurs selling touristy wares and working as cultural brokers. Evidently, although brandished in public rhetoric and targeted *en bloc* as though homogenous, *bumsters* are diverse and heterogeneous.

## Why do *bumsters* pursue female tourists?

Within the broader societal framework, the act of the less fortunate begging, requesting, demanding, or taking from those advantaged with more is intrinsic to everyday life. *Zakat* or almsgiving is among the five pillars of Islam. Giving charity over and beyond the alms is believed to bring favour before God and men. Beggars are fed by mosques and capable individuals every Friday after prayers, during the Ramadhan fast, and on Islamic holidays. Youths frequently offered to pay the public transport fares of elderly travellers unknown to them. Socio-cultural norms of respectability, reciprocity, responsibility and religiosity prescribe dependence on those perceived to be well-off, by those who are not. Thus it was common practice for rural kin and acquaintances to arrive unexpectedly and live for days on end with their urban connections, without contributing a cent towards their upkeep. One-way flows from the haves to the have-nots are established practice. They are the basis for most patronage relationships (see Ebron 2002).

Due to widespread unemployment and underemployment, many young men lack sustainable livelihoods and a stable source of regular income. Gender norms are tougher on men who are expected to mature into responsible providers *en route* to independence and eventual marriage. While it is socially acceptable for girls to depend on their family homes prior to marriage and husbands thereafter, a successful son contributes to the household, reproduces, supports his dependants, and ploughs resources back into his family and wider community (see Schroeder's 1996 discussion of the notion of useless husbands who relegate duties of provision to their wives). Providing a ram for annual Tobaski festivities is a masculine gender role that marks the men from the boys in a Muslim Gambian compound. It is also a measure of success. Returns from tourists cater for these demands. The mobility and agility of youthful masculine bodies enhances movement around in pursuit of income.

As Westerners, white tourists are perceived as the personification of wealth, prosperity and an endless solution to local lack. Their position – coming from the imagined West – seems to negate their humanness, reducing them to a big open purse. In resultant relationships (no matter how transient), the imagined inequalities between Westerner and local are paramount. Thus, tourists irrespective of gender pay for meals, entertainment, clothes, gifts, tips, transport fares and mobile-phone credit for the beach boy. Many *bumsters* reported preference of interacting with female over male tourists. Essentialist claims about women being more gentle, soft-spoken and easier to win over than men prevailed. Racialised and gendered justifications were offered:

White women are not loud and harsh like our black girls who can talk back, challenge and even shame you if you are not careful.

(Omar, focus group discussion, Kotu, 2005)

EBOU: If you keep on asking them about this and that, after a while you see their faces getting red because they want you to go away but you refuse. To send you away, a white woman will dip into her bag and give you *dalasis*. A man just walks away.

TIJAN: White women fear going out alone more than the men. They are the best for me, because if I give them a good time, guiding them here and there, they will appreciate it by giving a bigger tip. And if you get one outside the group tour, then you can even proceed to adult things.

(Focus group discussion, BB Beach, 2006)

The most frequently mentioned reason why *bumsters* chase female tourists centred around the hope of making a sexual connection, providing an addictive sexual experience, or simply falling in love and then carefully processing immigration to join the partner in the west. The sexual histories we compiled reveal both serial and multiple sexual relationships with tourists. The qualitative data highlight that most sexual relationships with tourists were short term and terminated with the tourist's departure back home. However, in some cases, there developed different measures of regularity ranging from permanence (illustrated by eight successful spousal unions), to short-lived marriages that broke up when the *bumster* migrated to the West, to returnee-tourists who reconnect with the same *bumster* (even though some of these women are married to men at home).

Migrating to the West was the ultimate dream of many *bumsters* because it carried the hope of leading to immense prosperity, and a well-paying job that would facilitate remittance sending to enable the male youth to fulfil his masculine obligations at home. Remittances are a mainstay for many households, communities, and local enterprises, including some developments in tourism. 'Going to The Western Union' is symbolic to earning income in local constructs and regular visits there boost social status. Many parents and siblings back home rely on the next remittance for their basic needs, thus many families do not condemn *bumster* aspirations because of the inherent financial potential.

Participants reported that while it was possible to receive remittances from male tourists, there was usually no reason for sustained giving between men.[9] However, there was widespread belief in possibilities to give (particularly older) female tourists unbridled sexual fulfilment enabling a link that the Westerners would want to nurture. Clearly these local narratives fit into racialised sexual fantasies, stereotypes and myths (see also O'Connell Davidson and Sanchez-Taylor 1999; Phillips 1999).

## Why the danger?

Why is *bumster* sexuality constructed as dangerous, thereby contributing to definitions of these male youths as a social problem? Unlike arranged marriages where families have an upper hand in choosing sexual partners, negotiating dowry, setting the schedule and advising the couple through culturally appropriate institutions of sexuality education, individual *bumsters* make the sexual choices in liaisons with tourists. The relationships are shrouded in secrecy, and often mystified. However, amidst wider economic challenges to their masculinity, the autonomy, risk, adventure, and self-actualisation in relationships with tourists are symbols of achieving self-styled manhood. *Bumster* sexuality avails opportunities to refashion local manhood in resistance to emasculation by economic hardships. Social and sexual connection with a Western tourist symbolises metaphors of power – be it wealth, age, race, geographic locus, and thereby rejuvenating possibilities. Personal narratives of *bumsters* seem to reverse Ebron's (2002:171) claim that such relationships threaten masculinity and 'feminize Gambian men'. Instead, *bumsters* report that when they consummate sexual relationships with 'powerful' Western women, their masculinity is strengthened. When the sexual connection leads to financial take-off and the ability to fulfil masculine roles, remittances are sent home which facilitate investments of diverse scale, and national development may be enhanced.

While Westerners may sexualise and eroticise the local Gambian men, the *bumsters* strategise, monetise and economise each encounter. Devoid of tangible commodities or pre-packaged professionalised services to offer tourists, *bumsters* thrive on interaction – whether social or sexual. Innovatively bending whichever way to meet tourists' every whim, they serve up companionship, conversation, negotiating local transport, price-cuts, proximity to 'the native', culture broking, translation, dance partner, escort, local knowledge, sexual services, relationship, partnership and business dealer. Providing sexual services is thus but one item out of a dense repertoire of possibilities. While exchange is integral to customary sexual behaviour in many African societies, the utility element does not sit well with outsiders who tend to liken it to prostitution.

Amidst widespread denial of HIV and AIDS as a local Gambian reality, we frequently encountered xenophobic distancing of the infection to outsiders. In this predominantly Muslim country, where premarital sex is forbidden and early and arranged marriages are widespread, it was common for participants to relegate HIV infection to foreigners, tourists, and expatriates. Interestingly, this local perception is in direct contrast to dominant Western perspectives that situate higher sexual risk among African host populations. In pursuit of deeper intimacy in their sexual activities with tourists, some *bumsters* reported it was necessary to overlook condom use which reportedly reduced pleasure. According to Bauer (2007:292) ' ... unfortunately unprotected sex with tourists (with unknown sexual histories) puts locals in a dangerous bridging position where infection can be transmitted to their local sex partners and to other tourists'.

However, protecting oneself against HIV infection was not a concern for the *bumsters* we interviewed. Some openly questioned the existence of HIV and AIDS within their immediate environs, arguing that they had never seen an HIV-infected person. Their multi-facetted and more immediate lack was more of a reality than HIV and AIDS. Some refrained from condom use as a strategy to communicate intimacy or a veneer of trust in their sexual relationships with tourists. It was clear that *bumsters* mainly obliged their tourist partners; thus if the tourist insisted on using protection during sex, it was so. Likewise if she preferred not to use condoms, the *bumster* played along in a bid to win her favour.

CHERNO: The condom is good for protection. But then if you ask her to use a condom she may think that you do not trust her enough or you think that she has got some sickness which she may spread to you.

TOURAY: Also, if you are thinking about winning her heart so she asks you to come to her home because of love, you have to make sex which is good. If you use that condom, she will not feel how powerful you are because the condom is just smooth-smooth sex.

(Focus group discussion, Manjai Kunda, 2005)

Condoms are not used by many of the boys on the beach when they are sexing *toubabs* because it will show that you do not trust the woman. Condoms spoil the plan of making a *toubab* trust you because the boys think that they can make her climax more if they go in without any thing disconnecting between their dicks and the woman. They call it dick-power. In our chats they say that that is what the *toubabs* come here to look for.

(Individual interview with Older Beach fruit seller)

Popular discourse about *bumsters* was infused with moralisations about generational decay because youths were forsaking local sexual practices and mimicking Western culture relayed through the media. In fantasizing about, pursuing and achieving sexual relations with female tourists, *bumsters* projected the image of local boys gone sour, thus they were commonly portrayed as spoilt, delinquent and mannerless. This was heightened when juxtaposed with images of brazen, strong, elderly women who were desiring agents willing to sexually interact with 'failed' youths. Ebron (2002:178) captures the tourists' portrayal: ' ... where the agency of women is supported and encouraged through a certain bravery, badness, and more blatant eroticism than what is allowed in "conventional" ideals of femininity'. *Bumster*–tourist relations thus assume the caption of degenerate sex, boundary transgression and risk.

In comparison to sex with local girls, however, there were ageist stereotypes of older foreign women being less pleasurable 'because their vaginas were wider and looser' (Maticka-Tyndale *et al.* 2005:36), their bodies were out of shape (Phillips 1999), or indeed carried the evidence of age such as wrinkles and saggy bosoms. Wagner (1986) discusses societal customs of intergenerational cross-gender interaction which are based on notions of respect, deference, distance and authority. However, by sharing social and sexual intimacy with older white strangers, *bumsters* invariably transgress these unwritten boundaries of propriety in the most polluting route: namely sexual activity. Evidently it is disconcerting to some segments in society, including the local women who are wives or sexual partners to these *bumsters*[10] thus the snide remarks, satire, abundance of lewd jokes and stereotypes about filthy delinquent *bumsters* and bumbling old white women (Jassey 2005).

This ethnographic study of *bumster*–tourist relationships in The Gambia disrupts the binary neatness of the analytical framework of exploitation within sex tourism. The notion of the First World exploiting the Third World is simultaneously confirmed and contested. Certainly these are often relationships of diverse inequalities. However, when exchange is mutual between *bumster* and tourist, who is to say that exploitation is present? If the fantasised sexual services of a black man are received in exchange for the dream of a plane ticket to an imagined West, who is exploiting who? Although the women tourists are often more economically advantaged, in negotiating a sexual relationship with the *bumster,* the women have to show a level of need for the *bumster* because he fulfils a particular void in their lives. Tact and care are vital in maintaining the balance between having (more than) sufficient material, financial or other support, and simultaneously lacking something – however vain, trivial or artificial – that only this *bumster* can provide. Transcending exploitation, perhaps locals and tourists who connect sexually for whatever duration, locate in each other mutual needs and negotiate reciprocal avenues of fulfilment. Rather than attempting to efface these sexual liaisons from public discourse, targeted policy and program development, it is important to open up spaces to further explore, contextualise and systematically bring on board actors' perspectives.

## Notes

1  This complexity is compounded by the January 2007 proclamations of the Gambian President that he possessed a cure for HIV/AIDS, which he subsequently administered to many HIV-infected individuals. The local popularity of the President's AIDS cure set back gains of the HIV/AIDS health education campaigns among the local population.
2  We conducted ethnographic fieldwork for 36 months between 2003 and 2007.
3  Pseudonyms are used to conceal identities.
4  A long-time resident of the Gambian coast, the second author has a history of diverse interactions with many *bumsters*. He facilitated entry into the study setting, and access to potential participants. An outsider to the Gambian context, the first author identified herself as an anthropology student researching sexual cultures of local youths. *Bumsters* often said this research provided them with an opportunity to 'air our side of the story'.
5  Attending a university education has long been a privilege of the wealthy.
6  Writing 25 years earlier, Harrell-Bond (1978:87) states, 'Truancy among school children has reached alarming proportions because the youngsters are on the beaches begging from tourists'.

7 The deception and manufacture of plight stories in order to effect profitable liaison was not the preserve of only males – however, reports about men abound more than they do women.

8 A sample of plots include: (a) an ill, divorced mother (with several dependant children) very recently suffered the roof of her mud hut blown apart in heavy rains. (b) A pregnant, widowed sister with three infants, who is suddenly admitted in hospital and needs expensive medications lest she or her unborn baby die. (c) Six orphaned younger siblings who are dependent on the *bumster* for school fees, shelter, clothes, food, health, etc., yet life is very hard because he just lost his full-time decent job and moved into a one-roomed house with all his dependants. (d) An intelligent sister who no longer studies because she was involved in a car accident that left her as an amputee. If only she could afford a wheelchair, her chances of resuming school will be restored.

9 Discussions of male–male sex tourism were constrained by social cultural criminalisation and stigmatisation of homosexuality in The Gambia on nationalistic and religious grounds.

10 Elsewhere (Nyanzi *et al.* 2005:566) we discuss how local sexual partners and spouses are not expected to be jealous of the *bumsters'* extramarital affairs, but rather be grateful for the potential opportunities arising out of sexual partnerships with tourists – particularly the imagined benefits of emigration to the West.

## References

Ashley, C., Goodwin, H.I., Boyd, C. (2000) *Pro-Poor Tourism: Putting Poverty at the Heart of the Tourism Agenda*. London: Overseas Development Institute.

Bauer, I. (2007) 'Understanding sexual relationships between tourists and locals in Cuzco/ Peru', *Travel Medicine and Infectious Disease*, 5(5): 287–94.

Brown, N. (1992) 'Beach boys as culture brokers in Bakau town, The Gambia', *Community Development Journal*, 27(4): 361–70.

Dahles, H., Bras, K. (1999) 'Entrepreneurs in romance: tourism in Indonesia', *Annals of Tourism Research*, 26(2): 267–93.

Department of State for Finance and Economic Affairs (2006) *Poverty Reduction Strategy: 2007–2011*. Banjul: DoSFEA.

Department of State for Education (2004) *Education Policy 2004–2015*. Banjul: DOSE.

Ebron, P. A. (2002) *Performing Africa*. Princeton: Princeton University Press.

Fleming, L. (2006) 'Gambian *bumsters* clean up their act'. *British Broadcasting Company News*. Online. Available from: www.news.bbc.co.uk/1/hi/world/africa/5383210.stm (accessed 17 June 2008).

Gambia Tourism Authority (2005) *The Gambia Tourism Development Master Plan – Draft Report*. Banjul: The Gambia.

Harrell-Bond, B. (1978) 'A window on the outside world, tourism and development in The Gambia', *American Universities Field Staff Reports No. 19*. Hanover, New Hampshire: American University Field Staff.

Jassey, K. (2005) 'In the eyes of the beholder: male and female agency in relation to "race", sexuality, love and money', Nordic Africa Days Workshop – *Sex and Gender in Africa: Critical and Feminist Approaches*. Uppsala.

Jeffreys, S. (2003) 'Sex tourism: do women do it too?', *Leisure Studies*, 22(3): 223–38.

Jennaway, M. (2008) 'Cowboys, *cowoks*, beachboys and bombs: matching identity to changing socio-economic realities in post 2005 North Bali', *The Asia Pacific Journal of Anthropology*, 9(1): 47–65.

Kempadoo, K. (2001) 'Freelancers, temporary wives and beach-boys: researching sex work in the Caribbean', *Feminist Review*, 67: 39–62.

Lawson, S., Jaworski, A. (2007) 'Shopping and chatting: reports of tourist-host interaction in The Gambia', *Multilingua*, 26: 67–93.

Maticka-Tyndale, E., Gallant, M., Brouillard-Coyle, C., Holland, D., Metcalfe, K., Wildish, J., Gichuru, M. (2005) 'The sexual scripts of Kenyan young people and HIV prevention', *Culture, Health and Sexuality*, 7(1): 27–41.

McCormick, N. (1994) *Female Salvation: Affirming Women's Sexual Rights and Pleasures*. Westport: Praeger.

Nyanzi, S., Rosenberg-Jallow, O., Bah, O., Nyanzi, S. (2005) '*Bumsters*, big black organs and old white gold: embodied racial myths in sexual relationships of Gambian beach boys', *Culture, Health and Sexuality*, 7(6): 557–69.

O'Connell Davidson, J., Sanchez-Taylor, J. (1999) 'Fantasy islands: exploring the demand for sex tourism', in K. Kempadoo (ed.) *Sun, Sex and Gold: Tourism and Sex Work in the Caribbean*. Lanham: Rowman & Littlefield Inc.

Oppermann, M. (1999) 'Sex tourism', *Annals of Tourism Research*, 26(2): 251–66.

Phillips, J. L. (1999) 'Tourist-oriented prostitution in Barbados: the case of the Beach Boy and the White female tourist', in K. Kempadoo (ed.) *Sun, Sex and Gold: Tourism and Sex Work in the Caribbean*. Lanham: Rowman & Littlefield Inc.

Ryan, C. (1999) 'Sex tourism: paradigms of confusion', in S. Clift and S. Carter (eds.) *Tourism and Sex: Culture, Commerce and Coercion*. London and New York: Pinter – 23–40.

Schroeder, R. (1996) '"Gone to their second husbands"': marital metaphors and conjugal contracts in The Gambia's female garden sector', *Canadian Journal of African Studies*, 30 (1): 69–87.

Shaw, M., Jawo, M. (2000) 'Gambian experiences with Stepping Stones: 1996–99', *PLA Notes*, 37: 73–78.

Taylor, J. S. (2006) 'Female sex tourism: a contradiction in terms?', *Feminist Review*, 83(1): 42–59.

UNAIDS (2007) *Gambia Country Profile*. Online. Available from: www.unaids.org/en/Regions_countries/countries/Gambia.asap (accessed 17 June 2008).

Van der Loeff, M. F. S., Sarge-Njie, R., Ceesay, S., Awasana, A. A., Jaye, P., Sam, O., Jaiteh, K. O., Cubitt, D., Milliga, P., Whittle, H. C. (2003) 'Regional differences in HIV trends in The Gambia: results from sentinel surveillance among pregnant women', *AIDS*, 17(12): 1841–46.

Wagner, U. and Yamba, B. (1986) 'Going north and getting attached: the case of Gambians', *Ethnos*, 51: 3–45.

# Chapter 9

# Fantasies, dependency and denial

## HIV and the sex industry in Costa Rica

*Jacobo Schifter and Felicity Thomas*

Since the 1990s, tourism has become a major part of Costa Rica's economy, with visitors attracted by the country's pristine beaches, stunning scenery and stable political climate. According to figures supplied by official sources at international airports, an estimated 1.9 million tourists visited Costa Rica in 2005, mainly from the USA and Europe (La Nacion 2005). Easy access from the USA and signs of a crackdown on sex tourism in parts of South East Asia have, since the 1990s, seen Costa Rica emerge as something of a new Mecca for sex tourism (Jimenez 1999; Seabrook 2001). As well as over 40 websites dedicated to promoting sex tourism in Costa Rica, sexual services are also promoted by hotels, travel agencies, and escort services and even by fishing trip promoters. Sex workers can be delivered to the client's hotel door in some towns. Clients can order a woman for an entire trip or one for every night at beach hotels. 'Didn't you like what was brought to you? *No hay problema*' says the information in one brochure, 'You can exchange her at no extra cost'.

Defining themselves as 'whoremongers' – often shortened to 'mongers', many of those travelling to Costa Rica are middle-aged US men who seek sex with young Latino women. As one man notes on an internet chatroom board aimed at sex tourists, the accessibility of Costa Rica's sex industry, based primarily in San José's 'Gulch' area, means 'I can get to CR for $313 right now. I can go to work ... work almost a full day. ... catch a non-stop after work and be banging a chica in the [Hotel] Del Buey by 10 pm that same night!'

Hotel Del Buey, Hotel El Duende[1] and others nearby are establishments in the Gulch that cater largely for sex tourists. The average occupancy rate for these hotels is 72 per cent. In a regular day, there are 667 occupied rooms, half of which are occupied by two men. This gives us approximately 1,000 persons per day. If the average stay in Costa Rica is seven days, there will be around 4,000 sex tourists per month and approximately 48,000 sex tourists per year in hotels in this area alone. Since there are many more hotels that cater to sex tourists and not all sex tourists stay in hotels, the maximum could be much higher, and may involve 5–10 per cent of the total number of visitors from the USA per year. If we add up this group with those US and Canadian ex-patriots who live in Costa Rica and who also participate in the sex trade, the numbers could double.

There is increasing recognition that the power relations involved in sex tourism are far from clear cut. Ryan and Hall (2001), for example, view sex tourism as an interaction between two groups of equally positioned yet marginalized people, while Kempadoo (2004) views tourists in the Caribbean as part of a dominating culture treated with respect by those in the sex industry (and often those in authority) for their role in providing an income to large numbers of people. Building on this work, we focus in this chapter on examining the complex and often contradictory motivations which influence both sex workers and sex tourists, and in so doing, offer an insight into the expectations, aspirations, fantasies and risks that underpin such relationships.

## Approach

Drawing upon the findings of an earlier study undertaken by the non-governmental organization the Latin American Health and Prevention Institute, research was undertaken in 2004 to map the sex tourism industry and gain insight into the characteristics and attitudes of the men who come to Costa Rica as sex tourists. Although sex work in Costa Rica is legal, pimping is not, and there was a considerable degree of difficulty in undertaking research involving either the owners of establishments known to sell sex or involving those purchasing sex. The main route by which information on sex tourists was gathered therefore was via internet forums which promote sex tourism in Costa Rica.[2]

Particular focus in this chapter is placed on the web forum *costaricaticas.com* which carries out a number of its own surveys and polls amongst its users.[3] The majority of the forum's users have internet identities, and do not reveal their real names. Other research methods involved identification and mapping of the most important sexual establishments in San José and in Jaco Beach on the Pacific coast of Costa Rica, in-depth interviews and focus groups with sex workers at three of these establishments, a count of condoms used in massage parlours and ethnographic observation.

### The sex workers

The mapping exercise found 543 sex workers and 219 tourists from the USA in 15 different sex establishments on one night in September 2004 during the slow tourist season in Costa Rica. Many of the sex workers who target tourists from the USA are not Costa Ricans but Colombian or Dominican women who have migrated to Costa Rica in search of improved social and economic opportunities. Almost two-thirds of the sex workers who are from Costa Rica have also migrated, in this case from rural areas to urban centres such as San José.

Importantly, migration, particularly for those coming from abroad, allows mothers, wives, girlfriends, or daughters a high degree of anonymity and protection from discrimination at home while also protecting their family from being associated with a 'loose' woman. However, rather than being forced into sex work through poverty, many come from low-middle class backgrounds and have some secondary education.

For some women, the appeal of raising a large sum of money in a relatively short period of time through sex work often underlies a move into the trade. Many of these sex workers are formally known as small-scale entrepreneurs who travel outside the country to purchase merchandise to sell in their home territory and/or in other countries. Women often rely upon sex work to build up their initial capital in order to begin a trading career in household goods or other items. They tend to leave sex work once the capital is accumulated. It is estimated by some informants therefore, that fewer than 20 per cent of the women are 'regulars'. Some of them come to work in the sex industry once a month and others only a few times each year. 'If I can't make enough at my beauty parlour,' says Mariana, 'I come here to make some extra bucks. I come to Del Buey only when I need cash'.

While women in Costa Rica work in the sex industry primarily for the money, it is not usually because they have no money in the first place. Most of the women already own a colour TV, a washing machine and a refrigerator. Some now want the latest mobile phone, a Gucci purse or a trip to Miami. María, for example, gets dressed at her home in one of the working class neighbourhoods that surround the capital city of San José. She works as a cashier during the day in Mas Por Menos, a large supermarket nearby making $250 a month. 'Not enough' she says, 'to live as I want'. María is not married and the two men who fathered her children disappeared from her life several years ago. To make ends meet and to be able to afford a car, she has another job at night. No one in her family or in her neighbourhood knows about her second profession, one that allows her to make three times as much money as a cashier at the supermarket. María is a sex worker who services tourists from the USA and works in one of the trendiest nightclubs and hotels in San José.

Interviews with sex workers, analysis of internet sex forums and ethnographic observation reveals that the migrant status of women from Colombia and the Dominican Republic enables them to enjoy particular advantages over the Costa Rican sex workers. They are reputed to live off sex work exclusively and invest accordingly with breast implants, fitness club memberships, expensive clothing and perfumes. Being 'pro' means they can be seen in restaurants, beach resorts, clubs and shopping malls with their clients while Costa Rican workers who live a double life and do sex work as a part-time job find it more difficult to be so exposed. They also tend to have more experience of living in an urban area which translates into better 'theatre' in seduction and in pleasing American men than Costa Rican sex workers, many of whom come from rural areas and are shy about certain sexual practices. They also tend to have a better command of English than Costa Rican sex workers which enables them to converse more easily with the sex tourists.

The incomes of sex workers have improved steadily in the past few years. In Hotel Del Buey, for example, the cost for one hour with a sex worker can range from US$100 to US$500 depending on the characteristics of the sex worker. The women who are deemed the most attractive can earn around US$1,000 to US$2,000 per night. Mexpat, a user of *costaricaticas.com* notes that 'high quality poontang in the Del Buey can get expensive. More and more chicas are asking US$100 an hour firm and some are coming off the top with US$200 or US$300 for a few hours or toda la noche'. Since pimps are not common in Costa Rica, most of this money is kept by the sex worker. Even those who are willing to negotiate down to US$80 an hour can pocket US$500 a night. The average income is around US$2,000 a week, not bad for a country where a professional makes around US$500 a month. The reason, according to Mexpat is because 'Unfortunately a lot of tourists are paying these prices which is just aggravating the problem'. The solution he sees is to look for cheaper street sex workers or workers in less prestigious establishments such as Casa Mila: 'Yes, there are still lots of very fine chicas who will go for US$50 or 20,000 colones', but, he laments, 'locating the ones who will go for this and give great service is tricky'.

Despite these rising prices, polls at the sex forums reveal that the majority of sex tourists spend under US$300 a day including sex. The average total expense of the trip according to Xanadu, a self-proclaimed expert from the sex forum, is around US$2,200. This includes sex with an average of 10 women at US$90 each, prices that are easily affordable for the average US sex tourist.

### The men

The average American man participating in the *costaricatica.com* sex forum is between 50 and 59 years of age (38 per cent). A smaller group is between 40 and 49 years of age (27 per cent). The rest is divided between the very young and the very old. Marylin, a sex worker, told me that the youngest man she has been paid to have sex with was a 13-year-old American boy introduced to her by his uncle at a private party in Guanacaste. The oldest man she had been with was 92 years old.

As to their physical appearance, 35 per cent of those polled in *costaricaticas.com* describe themselves as overweight, 31 per cent think that they are 'in shape', a similar percentage consider themselves to be 'average', and one percent think that they 'can't see their shoes'. One of the forum administrators who has met thousands of sex tourists provides this humorous, but not far from the truth, description of the typical monger:

(a) middle-aged, single and only meets American women with tons of baggage and problems not to mention saggy tits and baggy asses;
(b) older guys that had given up getting any sort of sex;
(c) married guys that want and need variety and want to feel young and viral [sic] again, i.e. looking for fountain of youth;
(d) single young guys frustrated with paying for expensive dates and getting no sex or very poor sex;
(e) guys that just like lots of sex and enjoy Latinas.

Sex tourists might generally be unattractive and old, but this does not mean they cannot find sex back home in the USA. On the contrary, many men report active sexual relationships with wives and partners at home. Nevertheless, when they talk about these sexual relationships, they claim to do it out of pity or pressure since they no longer feel attracted to wrinkles and saggy bodies. Happyman, for example, indicates that most mongers come to Costa Rica to get what is no longer attainable in the USA, that is, sex with beautiful women.

> Vegas Bob planted a statement in my head that I can't get rid of. He said, in his big loud voice, 'happyman, you will know you are not in CR when you go to the supermarket in the states and see a beautiful young girl behind the register … that you just love and gives you a roaring hard on … but, alas, you realize you can't have her. She is unattainable. That's when you'll know you are no longer in Costa Rica.'

Mongering seems to be a middle-class phenomenon. The sex forums are filled with posts from professional men with high incomes who appear to be highly educated and whose posts reveal insights and awareness of international politics and culture. It does not appear to be the typical working class guy who comes to Costa Rica for sex.

## The fantasy relationship

The forum participants are pretty open about the reasons why they look for paid sex. Some do not feel attractive enough to court young and beautiful women. Sixteen per cent admitted that one of the reasons for mongering is 'You are too hopelessly ugly to get laid at home'. The majority however, blame US women, who they perceive as aggressive, rude and not 'feminine'. In a poll taken at *costaricaticas.com*, 40 per cent responded that they come to Costa Rica because 'You hate *gringas* and love *Latinas* and only work at home to make money to go to Costa Rica and live'. According to Eljefe, men go to Costa Rica to fulfil their sexual desires without the ties and 'baggage' associated with relationships at home.

> We go to CR because we love to phuck, to fulfill our lust and fantasies – it's a quick-fix, an escape from our reality, the bitchy-cold wife/GF [girlfriend] or loneliness and everything else at home, the rush of leading a double life, with women that are so hot and sweet. And we can phuck all we want without all the complications and crap we'd normally have to put up with.

Why do they hate US women? LVSeve has been married three times; what he dislikes of them is 'having to pay for alimony'. PacoLoco advises everyone in the sex forums not to marry US women because he hates 'the band saw whine of anger, anger, anger that makes American women an international horror. It's there. It's real'. Dman agrees with him. He is still married but says if he had to do it again 'I would never ever marry again a *gringa*'.

CapoD2T claims to detest US women of his age because in spite of being 'well on the other side of their best day, [they] demand expensive dinners and wining and dining' and don't see themselves as 'dilapidated and with wrinkled faces' while Bombero claims simply that 'American woman are conniving, selfish, manipulating, dirty bitches'. Comments on the equal rights 'expected' by US women are also common in this abuse. At the same time, the men admit to being very attracted toward what they perceive as the flirtatiousness and warmth of Latin culture, factors which they also attribute to gender consciousness and patriarchal power hierarchies. As one user of *costaricaticas.com* wrote:

> Women's liberation, the feminist movement, and gay rights don't even exist [in Costa Rica]. ... If you're against this kind of thinking, you should forget about living in Latin America altogether because you'll run into a real brick wall as far as attempting to confront or change those customs is concerned and you will turn many of the Ticos against you.

Sex tourism in the Gulch therefore leads people to 'fantasy-land' where sex workers are perceived to be caring and easy to please, and partners back home are considered materialistic and selfish. Men who otherwise are smart, educated, business-savvy and quite insightful about life in the USA, become more like children in fairyland, surrounded by beautiful women who help them forget their real obligations back home. This exceptional time lived in the tropics is wonderful for relaxation and fun but it takes them to a mental state of denial that probably shields them from seeing the sex workers' real lives.

At the same time as the discussions on the internet forums suggest that men consider themselves to have a right to control the behaviour of Latina women, they also emphasise the men's desires to engage in romantic and loving relationships with the sex workers, spending time buying perfumes, flowers and chocolates, albeit so that they reassert a level of control over the relationship. Astroglide provides the following advice on love-making:

> Lesson #1: Teach them how to have sex your way. Spend time with them. Play the Magic CD. Light the candles. Lesson #2: Control the environment. Never let them watch TV. YOU set the mood and the atmosphere. That's why the candles and the CD are great ideas. It allows you to create a romantic mood, instead of just a banging and leave 'em experience.

This kind of 'girlfriend fantasy experience' is commonly reported on the internet forums and appears to be upheld in the actions of both the sex tourists and sex workers. This 'experience' has the intensity of a marriage but the shortness of a brief affair. It is not 'real' but it does make people act as if it was. The problem of this fantasy land is that you see no evil, including HIV.

## Denial, dependency and risk

Discussions on *costaricaticas.com* emphasise that many sex tourists locate HIV risk with what they perceive to be high-risk subgroups such as homosexuals, prisoners, Afro-Caribbeans and low-class sex workers. As such, they do not tend to associate their own behaviour as risky. As one user of *costaricaticas.com* states:

> Perhaps I am sticking my head into the sand on this issue, but I think distinctions must be made between various subgroups within the sex market. We are not all pedophiles, or gay or go with IV drug-using streetwalkers, or high-volume low rent local brothels.

However, while HIV prevalence rates in Costa Rica are relatively low for the region (estimated at 0.4 per cent of the adult population) they have shown a steady increase in the past decade (WHO 2008), and tourists and sex workers were reported to frequently engage in unsafe sex, and as such, increase risk of HIV transmission. As the following example suggests, one of the most common situations in which unsafe sex took place was in relationships in which the tourist's status had progressed from being a 'casual' to a 'regular' client:

> Jeff and María had such great sex that they dated several times. After the first night, they met again to go out for dinner, to dance and to have more sex. Jeff showed real interest in María's story of past sexual abuse and mistreatment by her father and husband number one. She in turn paid attention to his sad story of divorce and alimony payments that eat away his good salary in the States. During this second date, they would again have passionate sex and have more great conversations in Spanglish. Neither one is very sure that the other understands the story, but the attention seems real in both directions. Three days later, they are still having sex and it is still paid sex. María explained to Jeff that no matter how much she cares for him now, she still needs 'the dough' for her children. To prove her point, she makes two concessions: a reduction of the price for sex from $100 to $85 and an agreement to have sex without a condom.
>
> (Interview with María, sex worker)

As the above example demonstrates, sex workers' practices vary between casual and regular clients: a regular client is anyone who returns more than once. As such, the transition from a casual to a regular client is usually rather quick. A client might be casual on Monday night and a regular by Wednesday evening. Sex workers interviewed reported that they usually had control over the decision of whether to use a condom in these relationships. However, many were willing to have unprotected sex with these regular partners, particularly when this could result in additional gifts or incentives.

In cases, it was reported that sex tourists had 'married' (a term used here for falling in love with) sex workers, bought second homes for them to live in and sent them money.[4] When the man is in town, he acts as a lover and has a monopoly over the woman. When he leaves, she is 'free' to go back to her old job. According to the internet forum, men who set up a second house for their Costa Rican 'wife' expect intimate and bareback sex. As mentioned, however, anyone who becomes a regular client can also expect such services from the woman.

Ninety per cent of sex workers surveyed in 2000 said that they have had clients who do not want to use condoms. More than 60 per cent admitted having between one and nine casual clients who do not like to use them, a figure that is supported by more recent findings on *costaricaticas.com* which show that 49 per cent of the men had had unprotected sex with a sex worker in the past three years. Additionally, in this research, condoms were counted in trashcans in three of the most popular massage parlours on one day in 2004. Although it is not possible to know how many times each client had sex with one or more sex workers, nor the sexual practices clients engaged in, the fact that only 47 condoms were counted for 85 customers again suggests that high-risk sex is taking place.

These networks of HIV risk have multiple and transnational dimensions. The risk of HIV and other sexually transmitted infections involve the sex worker and her client, her 'married' partner, any 'real' partner she may have and any other sexual partner that any of these people may have. Prolijo's wife therefore might feel quite safe back in Florida with regard to HIV infection if she is unaware of her husband's relationships in Costa Rica. Similarly, Paco Loco's sexual partner, who works at Walmart in Kentucky, might never feel that she is part of an HIV risk group.

María explained that many of her customers missed the safe sex revolution in the 1980s and 1990s because they were in monogamous relationships back in the USA. The fact that 95 per cent of men polled claimed not to know anyone affected by HIV or AIDS suggests that they feel that it is not something that is likely to impact upon them. Discussions on the internet forums also show that many older men feel uncomfortable buying condoms, suggesting that they may also find it difficult to broach the subject with sex workers, particularly when only four per cent claim to be able to speak Spanish. It is not difficult to anticipate that they will face serious communication problems with women who are usually half their age and from a different culture, as well as fall into disagreements and disappointments over money, which may increase the chances of violent and unsafe sex. This kind of volatile relationship is further exacerbated by the widespread addiction to drugs and alcohol reported amongst sex tourists and sex workers in the Gulch.

Mongers admit that Costa Rica has become a sort of 'crack cocaine' that is hard to control. Don Gordo, for example, has made 59 trips to Costa Rica during the last decade; others have come more than 20 times. Alcohol, gambling and drugs have also become a major part of the dependency, not only for the mongers, but also for many of the sex workers. Rosaura, for example, admitted, 'Most of my money is wasted in gambling'. Lourdes, another sex worker, spends 50,000 colones a night in poker. José, a security guard at the Casino Del Buey, believes sex workers gamble half of their earnings, whilst it is known that many others are hooked to cocaine, alcohol and shopping.

Because of this spending, some sex workers owe street vendors and/or salesmen more than a month's income, meaning that they become increasingly reliant on sex work. María explains that being 'hooked' makes her feel 'out of control' and powerless. Lupe, a sex worker, feels she cannot control her unsafe sexual behaviour because she cannot stop her gambling habits. Miriam feels helpless with regard to alcohol, stating, 'I cannot stop drinking after my 10th drink. I don't remember what I do when I am drunk'. Part of the problem lies in the fact that sex workers are pressurized by bar owners to encourage their clients to purchase alcohol and in fact, women can make more money from these sales than from the sex itself. In-depth interviews revealed that sex workers not only found it difficult to control their own behaviour when drunk, but that alcohol made it increasingly likely that their clients would refuse to use condoms.

There is also a strong link between unsafe sex and cocaine consumption. From ethnographic observation it is clear that some sex workers use crack cocaine to lessen intoxication, in turn allowing them to consume more alcohol. This increasing need for cocaine forces them to spend more money on this drug and, accordingly, increases the need for more income from alcohol sales. This is a vicious cycle that leads them to make clients drink more and expose themselves to more pressures for having unsafe sex.

Another addiction among tourists from the USA, is to Viagra, Cialis and Levitra. According to the survey at *costaricaticas.com*, Viagra, called 'Vitamin V' is by far the most popular among sex tourists, taken to enable them to have sex with several prostitutes in a single day or for having sex for five hours in a row.

## Conclusions

The sex industry in Costa Rica is thriving as men travel from the USA and elsewhere to pursue relationships with young Latino women. Many of the women who become sex workers seek to increase their earnings and pursue what they perceive to be a more desirable kind of lifestyle, whilst the men travel to Costa Rica to seek the kind of fantasy relationship that they do not feel they can achieve in the USA.

Fantasies, dependency and denial can result in people engaging in multiple episodes of unprotected sex. Thus, while one of the tenets of sexual education in Costa Rica is the importance of honesty in negotiating safe sexual relationships this ideal is far removed from the reality of the Gulch and calls into question the relevance and use of traditional HIV educational and prevention interventions in Costa Rica.

## Notes

1 Names of hotels and bars have been changed to ensure anonymity.
2 A more detailed discussion of this research is available in Schifter-Sikora (2006).
3 Besides general interest for the web forum administrator and the sharing of information amongst users, the findings of the forum are not put to any other use.
4 According to the polls on *costaricaticas.com* 30 per cent of men claimed to be sending money to sex workers in Costa Rica.

## References

Jimenez, M. (1999) 'Costa Rica struggles with growing reputation as sex tourism Mecca', *Associated Press*, 28 November, 1999.

Kempadoo, K. (2004) *Sexing the Caribbean. Gender, Race, and Sexual Labor*, New York: Routledge.

La Nacion (2005) 'Aumento de turismo en 20%', *La Nacion*, 15 December, 2005.

Ryan, C. and Hall, M. (2001) *Sex Tourism and Liminalities*, New York: Routledge.

Schifter-Sikora, J. (2006) *Mongers in Heaven: Sexual Tourism and HIV Risk in Costa Rica and in the United States*, Lanham, Maryland: University Press of America.

Seabrook, J. (2001) *Travel in the Skin Trade: Tourism and the Sex Industry*, London: Pluto Press.

UNAIDS/WHO (2008) *Epidemiological Factsheet on HIV and AIDS: Core Data on Epidemiology and Response, Costa Rica, 2008 Update*. Online. Available from: www.who.int/globalatlas/predefinedReports/EFS2008/full/EFS2008_CR.pdf (accessed 29 October 2008).

# Chapter 10

# 'Que gusto estar de vuelta en mi tierra'

## The sexual geography of transnational migration

### Jennifer S. Hirsch and Sergio Meneses Navarro

Many Mexican migrants living in the USA return home annually to renew kin ties, jockey for social status and experience pleasure in their native land. These seasonal journeys represent a crucial shared reference point for local ideologies of gender, sexuality, and consumption as well as a vital factor shaping regional epidemiologies of HIV risk (Hirsch *et al.* 2007). In this chapter, we explore Mexican men's stories of homecoming, shedding light on how migration-related sexuality is negotiated within the moral and sexual geography through which Mexican migrants travel. We close with a discussion of the implications of these sexualized homecomings for the regional epidemiology of HIV and for HIV prevention.

The US Census Bureau estimates that in the year 2000 there were more than 20,000,000 Mexican-origin individuals in the USA, almost half of whom were foreign-born[1] – although it is hard to know for sure since a sizeable proportion of that population is undocumented. Circular labour migration between Mexico and the USA dates back at least to the late nineteenth-century Chinese Exclusion Act, which cut off the flow of Chinese workers and created a need for another source of low-cost labour for the expanding railroads of the American West. Since then, changing economic and political currents in the USA have produced some eras in which recruiters have penetrated deep into rural Mexico searching for able-bodied men and others in which US officials have rounded up and deported sizeable groups of Mexican-origin men, including even US citizens.

Migrants bring home more than dollars; recent evidence suggests that migration has been an important factor in the spread of HIV to rural, migrant-sending communities. The Mexican epidemic is primarily an urban gay epidemic, but the lower rural sex ratios and the large proportion of rural cases linked to migration suggests that in states such as Puebla, Guanajuato, Michoacan, Zacatecas and Jalisco there are important links between circular labour migration and HIV transmission; men get infected in the USA and then they return home to infect their wives (Hirsch *et al.* 2002; Bronfman and Leyva Flores 2008). In 2008, 350 thousand Mexicans are estimated to have migrated to the USA. The same year, return migrants were significantly over-represented among local

HIV-positive cases. In the states of Michoacán and Jalisco, for example, where 752 and 814 people, respectively, are infected with HIV, anywhere between one-quarter and a half of HIV cases occur among migrants and their family members, and across Mexico a growing proportion of HIV cases occur among migrants.

A great deal of attention has been paid to the sexual risks faced by labour migrants, both Mexican and otherwise, during their sojourns abroad. Migrants' vulnerability to HIV reflects the individual characteristics typical of many migrants, who tend overwhelmingly to be young men with little formal education and limited English skills. In addition, migrant men's vulnerability to HIV reflects the social characteristics of the communities in which they arrive, including generally more open norms about sexuality (in comparison to Mexico), the anonymity provided by being in a large urban context far from home, a lack of infrastructure to provide social support for migrants, exploitative working conditions, and a lack of access to health care (Magis-Rodriguez *et al.* 2004; Shedlin *et al.* 2006). Little has been written, however, about return migration and sexual risk. We take up that topic here, locating it within a broader discussion of the gendered sexual geography through which migrants navigate on both sides of the border.

## Fieldsite and methods

Degollado, with a population of about 15,000, is the *cabecera municipal* or county seat. It hums with commerce on most mornings, as townspeople go about their business and residents of outlying agricultural communities come into town to shop, wait in line to see the Presidente Municipal, visit an internet café, or pick up money sent from the north. Located in Western Mexico about 90 miles east of Guadalajara, Degollado has a long history of labour migration to the USA. Early in the twentieth century, men from Degollado helped build the railroads in the American West. Their sons, born in the 1930s and 1940s, journeyed north as temporary labour migrants under the *Bracero* programme to work in the fields of the Salinas Valley or the factories of Chicago. As is true more generally, more recent generations of migrants from Degollado journey beyond the traditional gateway cities of Chicago and Los Angeles to work in North and South Carolina, Georgia, and Tennessee, where the shifts in the US population have created great demands for manual labourers in construction and food service.[2] Those lining up in the plaza in the early dawn hours to take a bus which somehow (mysteriously, given their lack of entry visas) deposits them safe on the other side of the border are the granddaughters as well as the grandsons of the Bracero-era migrants; although a stint in the north poses risks (both imagined and real) for young women beyond those faced by young men, the Degollado migration stream has demonstrated the same feminization as in other migration streams throughout Mexico (Cerrutti and Massey 2001). For young men seeking to marry and establish their own homes, however, temporary labour migration remains a nearly obligatory rite of passage since young men in rural Western Mexico lack other options for economic mobility (or even survival).

Data for the present study were collected during two separate fieldwork periods. The first, in 1995 and 1996, consisted of 15 months split between Degollado and Atlanta (see Hirsch, 1998; Hirsch 2003), exploring generational and migration-related changes in marital ideologies and in sexual and repro- ductive health practices. The main method for data collection was life history interviews, collected from a matched sample of 13 pairs of women: half were in Degollado and a nearby agricultural community, with the matches comprised of their sisters and sisters in law who were living in Atlanta. These interviews were supplemented by participant observation and interviews with some women's mothers and husbands. Men's extramarital sexual practices were not a central concern, but as a result of an interest in migration's influence on marriage it was possible to learn a good deal about the ways in which symbolic aspects of transnational social space shapes sexual practices. The second fieldwork period, from January to June and December of 2005, was conducted in collaboration with Sergio Meneses, a Mexican colleague, as part of a multi-site comparative study exploring the social factors that put married women at risk for HIV infection (Hirsch *et al.* 2007; Hirsch *et al.* 2009). We used marital case studies, participant observation of domestic and social life, archival research, and key informant interviews to learn about men's participation in commercial sex. Since Sergio could directly observe men's socializing, we learned a significant amount about those practices.

## Return migrants and the search for authentic pleasures

In return for months as submissive and obedient workers in the North, migrants returning home in November and December hope to be welcomed home as conquering heroes. Suitcases bulging with gifts and pockets (for the lucky ones) full of dollars, they seek three things in exchange for their generosity: gratitude (which legitimates the risks taken and the pleasures foregone in the north and creates their social personhood in Mexico through the maintenance of kin ties); social status (the pleasure of having enough to give, and of having others know it); and the production of an authentically Mexican good time. The flourishes of *mexicanicidad*, Mexican-ness, are everywhere this time of year: corn kernels sit overnight soaking to be made into pozole; the fat mariachis in the plaza polish up the silver buckles on their pants and get to work; the 'Aztec' dance troupes in town rehearse feverishly, readying their *trajes típicos* (typical costumes), and their ankle bands with shells, and women who buy tortillas the rest of the year go to the mill early to grind corn for fresh hot homemade ones. Part of the effort is visual, accomplished through the splendour of the plaza and the parade during the fiestas; part of it is relational, experienced through the (genuine) love and warmth of those from whom they are so far most of the year; and part of it takes material form in the patterns of status-oriented consumption so evident during the migrants' return.

One of the key material results of these vast flows of migrant wealth is the transformation of Degollado into a town that looks Mexican – in the same way that the Japan Pavilion at Disney's Epcot centre 'looks' Japanese.[3] The oldest buildings in Degollado, dating back to the early nineteenth century, are built of thick blocks of local stone with elaborate ironwork windows and spacious inner courtyards. More commonly, however, the many buildings constructed during the town's rapid (remittance-funded) growth over the past four decades are made of cement, steel, and brick, faced with or decorated by *cantera*, the sandstone carved in local workshops on the edge of town. Cantera trims balconies, windows, balconies, doorframes, and downspouts; it screams money in a way that would be appreciated by a Dutch burgher or a dot-com millionaire. Migrants recreate their home communities to be the hometowns they wished they had had, paving the plaza, painting the church, buying the fireworks, and paying for the rides (see also Smith 2006). In 2004, during the December holidays, for example, the migrants collected enough money so that the rickety carnival rides in the plaza could be free for all school-aged children during the day they were honoured at Mass – a potent symbol for all of the way that migrants' munificence laid the material foundation for the shared pleasures of the plaza at night.

## The sexual geoscapes of a transnational community

The north is a land of moral peril as well as a key source of economic status. Any story about someone who has transgressed local sexual norms – whether through a flamboyantly public homosexuality, through a pre-marital pregnancy, or through a poorly managed extramarital affair – is likely to end with the refrain, '*y luego se fue para el norte*' (and then he (or she) went to the USA). This was the case with the woman who owned the pizzeria across the street from Doña Evita's house, who during my most recent visit was found by her husband in bed with her lover. It was also true of Pablito the flower store owner, who during my first stay in Degollado would mince by daily, stopping to wink at Evita's handsome son. The constant flow north of those who do not fit in locally only serves to reinforce the vision of the USA as a land where anything goes – indeed, ethnographic work on sexuality among migrants has suggested that people's own repertoires and desires may shift in response to this supposedly more liberal sexual climate (Bronfman *et al.* 1998). Combined with US-made movies and dubbed-into-Spanish versions of *Baywatch*, reports of licentiousness across the border are a vital part of the local sexual imaginary.

Migration is an economic rite of passage and a key step into adulthood (Hirsch 2003) but young men also see a chance to taste some of the pleasures of 'loose American girls' – who, as one young woman in Degollado told me, 'go through men like Kleenex' – before coming home to marry a respectable girl from a local family. Men who have been '*al otro lado*' delight in recounting their exploits and triumphs; the pleasure they take is not merely the carnal delight in the flesh, but also the perverse delight of screwing the citizens of a country that has screwed them – and their forebears – in so many ways, so that their triumphs read like symbolic reconquests of American territory. This eagerness to taste foreign meat intersects with the greater availability of casual sex partners in the USA. In Degollado, sex with a local girl incurs a whole set of expectations and obligations. The combination of American women who are (relatively) more independent as sexual agents, the easy availability of commercial sex and the desperate loneliness many migrants feel as they navigate through life far from home, all contribute to the notion of a country in which anything goes. As the older generation says, nodding their heads disparagingly, '*no es libertad, es libertinaje*' (it's not freedom, it's licentiousness).

Racialized notions of beauty create another layer in the erotics of migration; the persistent Mexican phenomenon of *Malinchismo*, a sort of ingrained self-deprecation of all things Mexican and a concomitant preference for the foreign, the northern, and the blonde, makes young men that much more eager to have sex with the fair-skinned 'beauties' that tempt them.[4] Despite the fair skin of some Degollado residents, girls with blue eyes and naturally blonde hair would be beyond the reach of most labour migrants, so the lure of bedding '*una rubia de categoría*' or high-class blonde (the phrase is actually the tag-line for a beer marketing campaign that plays on the pun between a light beer and a light-haired girl) is just one more aspect of the temptations that await in the north. This fascination with light hair holds true regardless of the actual comeliness of the maiden in question; Josefina's son in Wisconsin proudly sent home a picture of his common-law *gringa* wife, who all agreed was extraordinarily ugly, so that his mother and siblings could see how fair she was.

Migration as a sexual rite of passage plays out somewhat differently for girls. Gendered hierarchies of sexual prestige, expressed in the local saying '*el hombre no pierde nada, la mujer pierde todo*' (men don't lose anything, women lose everything [through sex]), keep women from screwing their way across America – or, at least, from bragging about it. Mexican social constructions of sexuality emphasize appearance rather than actual behaviour; adolescent girls (or at least some of them) may be equally eager for gringo flesh but they certainly know that talking about it back home will do nothing to enhance their reputation or marriageability. When women come back and show off about having been in the USA, they preen about gendered patterns of consumption – beauty products, home appliances, sales at the mall – but not about sex.[5] In ways both licit and illicit, this is the landscape of sex: women flee – or are banished from – Degollado as punishment for misbehaviour; men go seeking their fortune (and easy sex) but then come home looking for a nice girl to marry; their nice girl may have been two-timing them the whole time under the assumption that there is no sure thing. (This two-timing is so common that there is a local phrase for it; young men talk about 'pedalling someone else's bicycle'.)

## Coming home

What migrants do and buy when they return home takes on deeper meanings when seen in the light of what home means, and what it has meant to them to be away. Women returning as migrants use their money to flaunt their success, but they do so through the cultivation of their own bodies – adorning them with expensive jewellery, clothes, and cosmetics, and even engaging in exotic foreign practices such as aerobics and pilates – rather than through the conquest of others' bodies. Migrant men's status-oriented consumption includes heavy gold jewellery (among proponents of the *cholo* look), expensive cars, trucks and four wheeled all terrain vehicles, the building of homes, and of course gifts for their families, but our primary interest here is sex and, to a lesser extent, the alcohol that smoothes the way. In the cantina, when men pay for rounds of drinks in December, Sergio would sometimes see them take out their billfolds, which inevitably were double; on one side, the pesos neatly folded, with dollars on the other. No one actually pays in dollars, but paying for a round of drinks becomes an opportunity to flash a wad of cash, to show others how well you did in the north.

In December of 2004, for example, Sergio showed up at one of the town's more expensive bars around nine pm. The Terraza, on the second floor of one of the colonial-style buildings ringing the plaza, is distinguished from the grungier cantinas on the outskirts of town not just by location or price but also by the fact that it is a place where it is increasingly common to see respectable young women drinking in public, either with their boyfriends or even, occasionally, in all female groups. Sergio fell into a conversation with four men: Felipe, Juan, Diego, and Pancho. They were all dressed in the ranchero style and in their mid-30s, and looked to him to be a bit effeminate. Juan, Sergio knew, had a reputation as a closeted homosexual. Diego and Pancho had recently arrived from the USA. The fourth, Felipe, was an older married man who has legal residence in the USA, who owns four restaurants *al otro lado*, and who seemed quite intent that evening on getting it on with one of Sergio's friends, a young woman, who was at the same table with them early on in the evening. Throughout the evening, Felipe's refined tastes showed his companions how successful he had been in the USA; he drank nothing but Don Julio tequila, quite dear at more than 10 dollars for each small glass.

After the bars closed in Degollado, the five of them set out for Los Pelícanos, a table dance club about 20 kilometres away, in Juan's shiny new pickup, stopping first to fortify themselves at one of the taco wagons around the plaza – and to pick up another bottle of Don Julio for the road. As Sergio later told it, the ride sounded terrifying. Juan was quite drunk, it was dark and had been raining all day, and the twisty 20 kilometres between Degollado and La Piedad was already lined with white crosses marking those who did not quite make it. Upon entering Los Pelícanos, Don Felipe called to the host to bring them five women to sit on their laps, *una para cada cabrón, para que se hagan hombres* (one for each asshole, to make them into men). In spite of being somewhat overwhelmed by both the weight and closeness of his own companion, Sergio observed, as he wrote later in his fieldnotes, how they eagerly caressed – and were caressed by – their hired girlfriends:

> I see that Juan is staring with seriousness and shock at the enormous breasts of the woman who cosies up to him and wiggles her bottom. Her hands sweep over the nervous cowboy's penis, through his pants, and it looks like he has an erection. Diego's hands are everywhere: her butt, her boobs, her legs, her neck, and he even seems to be sticking several fingers into her vagina. Felipe is talking, very seriously and with eyes of devout love, to the woman who costs him two hundred pesos every five or ten minutes. She listens to him with care.

Diego buys a ticket to go with his companion into a curtained side room. For 150 pesos (about $13.50 in US dollars), one ticket buys a man one song's worth of time, supposedly for a private strip tease. If he buys several tickets together, the time allows for pleasures beyond the merely visual. As Sergio writes,

> Diego takes about twenty minutes and he comes back very happy. He says that '*que cogió muy sabroso*' (they had a great fuck) – and then he looks at the ethnographer and says, 'but I did use a condom, OK? Even though these chicks are very clean.'

Several hours and bottles of tequila later, the bill came to more than nearly US $400. Don Felipe proudly whipped out a billfold, only to find – sheepishly – that he had drunk himself down to his last 2,800 pesos. The other four chipped in to cover the remainder. At three thirty am, they head back; Sergio, as the least drunk, was delighted that they accepted his offer to drive back. Sergio drops Don Felipe and Pancho off at their respective homes, and then tries to rouse Diego and Juan, sleeping in the back, to find out where they live. Finding his efforts to be fruitless, he gives up, parks the truck, tucks the keys in Juan's front jacket pocket, and leaves them sleeping in the car to walk back to his house in the quiet hour before dawn.

These scenes are repeated throughout the year but with a particular intensity during the winter months, the season of migrant return. That is the season when dollars from the north come to buy sex in the south, when the crush of cars with gringo plates in the strip clubs outside of La Piedad is particularly heavy, and when the marriages arranged during the previous year's courtship season are celebrated by one last night with the strippers and the guys. Los Pelícanos marks the middle range economically; certainly not an inexpensive evening on the town, but nowhere near the 2,000 pesos (at the time, around $200 US) that Andres would brag about paying (just for himself) at his favourite place in Guadalajara. At this luxurious pleasure dome, men can choose from an assortment of supposedly gorgeous, slender women from a variety of Eastern European nations, who provide an invigorating massage and a blow job in tastefully appointed settings. At the other end of the spectrum lies the red light district in nearby Atotonilco, about 20 minutes west of town along the highway towards Guadalajara. Here, down a sad alley to which one buys access from a policeman standing guard (who, ironically, gives out receipts that merely say *obras públicas* (public works)), lie many small grimy bars, including the Bar Degollado, eponymously named for the hometown of its many working class patrons. Here the price of a quickie, no condom required, ranges from 100 to 200 pesos.

Men choose to celebrate their homecomings in this way for many reasons – not just, as a naturalizing explanation would suggest, because it feels good and their wives cannot stop them. The task of anthropology is to make the familiar strange; it should not be any more obvious to us that men choose to show off their hard-earned wads of dollars through buying sex than it was to Malinowski that the Trobrianders measured status through pigs and yams – or that these men's wives choose to buy gold, rather than men, when they return to their native land.

Turning this hard-earned money into shared pleasure is an assertion of their humanity, of their commitment to a different metric of social value. In the USA, many Mexicans say, people live to work, whereas in Mexico people work so that they can live. Felipe was celebrating the return to a space that values pleasure and experience for its own sake, his temporary escape from the relentless economic rationality of life in the USA. These men are free, for the moment, from the ruthless rules of a foreign land, from the constant fear of deportation, from an unintelligible language, from a protective stance of being *agachado* (humble and bent down). As I chatted with a restaurateur whose primary residence is in the USA, at his niece's fifteenth birthday party on his family farm outside Degollado, for example, he described how he exercises in each place: in his suburban US home, he keeps fit by running on a treadmill in the basement, whereas back on the farm in Degollado he hikes daily at sunrise, delighting in the dawn sounds of birds and animals, watching the rosy glow spread through the sky as his neighbours return from the first milking. In the USA, he continued, communication is purely instrumental; people talk just to say what is necessary for business. During the months at home, in contrast, he can spend the whole evening in conversation with a friend or relative, talking just for the pleasure of companionship, without once looking at his watch.

These men, however, are not just celebrating being home – they are celebrating returning home *as men*. Their dalliances are not just about physical pleasure but about the pleasure of power – the power of being away from the *migra*, away from their bosses and from their *jefas* (the female term for boss is used with affection to denote wives and mothers), of being away from seatbelts and drunk driving laws and the tiny crowded apartments in which they live to be able to save their money *para gozarlo* (to enjoy it), when they return home. Roger Rouse (1991) has written about the emasculation experienced by temporary labour migrants, who are stripped of the gendered access to mobility which is such a key privilege of Mexican masculinity, because the danger of everyday life in the USA forces them to spend as little time as possible in the street. Men's florid displays of Mexicanness at home (cowboy hats, boots, large belt buckles) can be seen as a pouring forth of all that which they hid behind workboots and baseball caps during the long months in the North, hoping not to stand out, not to call attention to themselves. Men's casual sexual liaisons – represented here by Diego's enthusiastically roving hands – reflect this same assertion of mastery of all that surrounds them.

These long boozy evenings are also about the pleasure of affect, of *cariño*, of the touch of a true friend and the ear of someone who cares deeply – but this affect is shared not between men and their hired girlfriends but among the men themselves. The sex is almost incidental; the main project during these evenings is the construction and enjoyment of deep social and emotional bonds between men. The women may neutralize the almost sexual charge of intimacy, the way an arm around the shoulders threatens (or promises?) to turn into a deep and passionate kiss between two men with moustaches. Organizing these outings around sex with women, ironically, keeps them safe from women, as the only women allowed into the charmed circle are those who men invite – and can dismiss at will – a much less complicated and intrusive presence than that of the women whose beds and tables they share during their daily lives. These all-male spaces, of which the cantinas, bars, and table-dance lounges described here are prototypical, are hothouses for the propagation and nurturing of homosociality, which is both a central feature of Mexican daily life and a channel through which resources are distributed and negotiated. Deals are made, bonds are forged or broken, *compadres* are chosen, and life goes on, one tequila at a time, as men breathe a deep sigh of relief, secure in the knowledge that they are finally home.

## And HIV?

Admonitions telling migrants to be faithful are likely a waste of time; sexual adventuring is so deeply woven into the fabric of migration that we might speak of the sexual organization of society for migrants rather than the social organization of migrant sexuality (Parikh 2007; Smith 2007; Hirsch *et al.* 2007; Wardlow 2007; Phinney 2008). Community-level interventions need to address the social – and homosocial – nature of extramarital sex, providing other ways for migrants on both sides of the border to fill their affective needs. It seems beyond the possibilities of even the ablest social engineering to create community-level interventions for returning migrants which can compete with the allure of Los Pelícanos – but it would certainly be possible to improve upon the very limited options for diversion available to Mexican migrant men in the USA. Loneliness and alienation play an important role in driving migrant men to seek sex while they are far from home (Hirsch *et al.* 2009). For those who are not interested in praying or playing soccer, there are few diversions other than dollar dance halls, strip clubs, and a few minutes with a shared sex worker. Community-level interventions – expanded hours for libraries (which provide migrants free access to computers so they can email with family back home), gyms, pool halls, fixing up old cars, and other recreational spaces, English classes, and other opportunities for continuing education – could provide alternative forms of entertainment. A less restrictive migration regime would make undocumented workers less afraid of spending time outside engaged in open-air recreation, and migration reform might even enable families to migrate together (which might reduce, although not eliminate, men's interest in seeking sex while in the USA).

For those who prefer the Church to the soccer field, faith-based programmes might serve to interrupt the migration-HIV risk nexus. The Catholic Church is the pre-eminent social institution bridging transnational communities, and it might be possible to use this existing power, coupled with Mexican Catholicism's embrace of embodied suffering as an expression of religious devotion, to develop a new sort of invented tradition, in which Mexican men commit to abstinence – or at least managed infidelities – in a parallel to that paradigmatic moment of embodied suffering and the deliberate abstention from pleasure, Jesus' encounter with the devil in the wilderness. The Church is, after all, led by men who commit themselves to a lifetime of controlling their own desires for the good of the greater community.

Extramarital sex on both sides of the border is a structural aspect of social organization; the fundamental cause here is not an underdeveloped Mexican masculinity but rather an overdeveloped US taste for the good life on the cheap – only possible because of the flow of migrant labour. These situations of HIV vulnerability are created by the migration regime, and so the most powerful interventions will be at the ballot box and in the halls of Congress. In the USA, the migration-HIV nexus ought to figure in conversations about migration policy, since the long separations of workers from their families play such a prominent role in shaping migration-related risk. When, as with Mexican workers in the USA, migrants are seen as disposable bodies, sort of cannon-fodder in the global wars of capitalism, many opportunities for primary prevention, for HIV testing, and for access to care are missed because the jobs at which migrants work provide no health care. Similarly, when migrants are shunted off into trailers, crammed into company shacks, or crowded into neighbourhoods with little in the way of public services, the absence of any explicit policy to create opportunities to build human capital accounts to a de facto community development policy of deliberate underdevelopment. In none of these situations is there an explicit policy goal of creating HIV risk for migrants. However, by not acknowledging that the *con la mano de obra viene un cuerpo y un corazón* (that labour is rendered by humans with complex needs) – the result is essentially an implicit policy that permits this situation. In all of these situations, the relatively low price of goods and services provided through migrant labour is predicated upon a hidden cost – the cost of sexual and HIV risk, borne not by the company that takes the profit, nor by the consumer who enjoys the product, but by the labourer who produced it.

## Notes

1 American Factfinder Fact Sheet on the Mexican Population, drawn from 2000 census data, available from: www.factfinder.census.gov/home/saff/main.html?_lang=en (accessed 14 November 2008).
2 Durand, Jorge, Massey, Douglas S., and Charvet, Fernando. *Social Science Quarterly* (University of Texas Press); 2000, Vol. 81, Issue 1, pp. 1–15.
3 Epcot Center is one of the amusement parks at Disneyworld in Florida. A visit to Epcot provides an opportunity to 'to celebrate the fascinating cultures and wonders of the world' through pavilions showcasing the cuisines and handicrafts of Mexico, Norway, China, Italy, Germany, Japan, Morocco, France, the USA, and Canada. www.disneyworld.disney.go.com/wdw/parks/parkLanding?id=EPLandingPage (accessed 25 September 2008).
4 Colour is frequently a marker of class in Mexico, but in this particular region of Mexico (Los Altos de Jalisco) the issue is further confused by the relative common-ness (compared, say to Southern or Eastern Mexico) of people with fair skin, green or blue eyes, and light brown or even blonde or red hair. Locals proudly claim that this colouring is so common because the region was settled by the French who were (supposedly) much more prone to kill the indigenous people rather than to reproduce with them, but regardless of the actual source of the local physiotypes, it is true that some in Degollado resemble their northern neighbours much more than their southern ones. However, the use of physiognomy to mark social class persists, so that, for example, lighter colour facilitates marrying up.
5 Not only did Mexican women seem on the whole relatively uninterested in American men, but in fact on more than one occasion I fielded questions about my own sex life, particularly regarding how frequently my husband and I have sex, asked with the intention of bolstering these women's assumptions (presumptions) that those pale and overly cerebral men in the north cannot possibly be as virile as their own men are.

## References

Bronfman, M. and Leyva Flores, R. (2008) 'Migración y SIDA en México', in Córdova Villalobos, J. Á., Ponce de León Rosales, S. and Valdespino, J. L. (eds) *25 años de SIDA en México. Logros, desaciertos y retos*. México: Secretaría de Salud, CENSIDA e Instituto Nacional de Salud Pública.

Bronfman, M., Sejenovich, G. and Uribe, P. (1998) *Migracion y SIDA en Mexico y Central America [Migration and AIDS in Mexico and Central America]*. Mexico: CONASIDA.

Cerrutti, M. and Massey, D. S. (2001) 'On the Auspices of Female Migration from Mexico to the United States', *Demography*, 38: 187–200.

Hirsch, J. S. (1998) *Migration, Modernity and Mexican Marriage: A Comparative Study of Gender, Sexuality and Reproductive Health in a Transnational Community*. Baltimore, Maryland: Johns Hopkins University.

—— (2003) *A Courtship after Marriage: Sexuality and Love in Mexican Transnational Families*. Berkeley, California: University of California Press.

Hirsch, J. S., Higgins, J., Bentley, M. E. and Nathanson, C. A. (2002) 'The Social Construction of Sexuality: Marital Infidelity and Sexual Transmitted Disease-HIV Risk in a Mexican Migrant Community', *American Journal of Public Health*, 92: 1227–37.

Hirsch, J. S., Meneses, S., Thompson, B., Negroni, M., Pelcastre, B. and del Rio, C. (2007) 'The Inevitability of Infidelity: Sexual Reputation, Social Geographies, and Marital HIV Risk in Rural Mexico', *American Journal of Public Health*, 97: 986–96.

Hirsch, J. S., Muñoz-Laboy, M., Nyhus, C. M., Yount, K. M. and Bauermeister, J. A. (2009) They Miss More Than Anything Their Normal Life Back Home: Masculinity and Extramarital Sex among Mexican Migrants in Atlanta , *Perspectives on Sexual and Reproductive Health*, 41(1): 23–32.

Hirsch, J. S., Smith, D. J., Wardlow, H., Parikh, S., Phinney, H. and Nathanson, C. A. (2009) *The Secret: Love, Marriage, and HIV*. Nashville, Tennessee: Vanderbilt University Press.

Magis-Rodriguez, C., Gayet, C., Negroni, M., Leyva, R., Bravo-Garcia, E., Uribe, P. and Bronfman, M. (2004) 'Migration and AIDS in Mexico: An Overview Based on Recent Evidence', *Journal of Acquired Immune Deficiency Syndromes*, 37: S215–26.

Parikh, S. (2007) 'The Political Economy of Marriage and HIV: The ABC Approach, "Safe Infidelity", and Managing Moral Risk in Uganda', *American Journal of Public Health*, 97: 1198–208.

Phinney, H. M. (2008) '"Rice Essential, but Tiresome, You Should get Some Noodles": the Political Economy of Men's Extramarital Sex and Married Women's HIV Risk in Hanoi, Vietnam', *American Journal of Public Health*, 98: 650–60.

Rouse, R. (1991) 'Mexican Migration and the Social Space of Postmodernism', *Diaspora*, 1: 8–23.

Shedlin, M. G., Drucker, E., Decena, C. U., Hoffman, S., Bhattacharya, G., Beckford, S. and Barreras, R. (2006) 'Immigration and HIV/AIDS in the New York Metropolitan Area', *Journal of Urban Health-Bulletin of the New York Academy of Medicine*, 83: 43–58.

Smith, D. J. (2007) 'Modern Marriage, Extramarital Sex, and HIV Risk in Southeastern Nigeria', *American Journal of Public Health*, 97: 997–1005.

Smith, R. C. (2006) *Mexican New York: Transnational Lives of New Immigrants*. Berkeley, California: University of California Press.

Wardlow, H. (2007) 'Men's Extramarital Sexuality in Rural Papua New Guinea', *American Journal of Public Health*, 97: 1006–14.

# Chapter 11

# From migrating men to moving women

## Trends in South Africa's changing political economy and geography of intimacy

*Mark Hunter*

Since the 1940s when Sidney Kark (1949) wrote his famous article 'The Social Pathology of Syphilis' male migration has remained a prominent explanation for high rates of sexually transmitted infections in Southern Africa. Kark's landmark piece outlined how rural-born 'African' men moved to the distant gold or diamonds mines for long periods, became infected with syphilis and then returned to infect their rural partner(s).[1] As AIDS came to the fore in the 1980s, this model appealed to many constituents. Yet I outline here a number of relatively recent but vitally important trends that affect intimacy, namely rising unemployment and social inequalities, dramatically reduced marital rates, and the extensive geographical movement of women as well as men in contemporary South Africa. Methodologically, this approach combines political economy, geography, and ethnography and key institutions it addresses are the labour market and the household.[2]

The complex interplay between race, class, and geography belies a single new model of migrancy or a single political economy of intimacy; what follows in this chapter is schematic and suggestive. There are several other caveats that must be made. This paper mainly considers poor South Africans and specifically those classified as 'African' under apartheid. It also considers only one side of the political economy of sex, namely sexual relationships between men and women; it does not look at the connection between political economy, same-sex relationships and HIV or, indeed, sexual violence and AIDS.[3] Furthermore, as many have powerfully argued, AIDS and sex are not the same thing: racialized assumptions can exaggerate the importance of sex to the spread of HIV and exoticize sexuality in problematic ways (see Vaughan 1991 and McClintock 1995 on racial tropes surrounding African sexuality and Stillwaggon 2006 for a recent reassertion of the significance of nutrition, parasites and other co-factors in HIV transmission in Africa).

That said, nationally, between 1990 and 2005, HIV prevalence among pregnant women in South Africa jumped from less than 1 to around 29 per cent.[4] And the fact that millions of dollars worth of intervention campaigns have had seemingly little effect demands that more attention be paid to the structural roots of the epidemic. This chapter builds on a now fast-growing and rich literature on the political economy of intimacy in the context of HIV and AIDS (for instance Farmer 1999; Schoepf *et al.* 2000; Hirsch and Wardlow 2006; Padilla *et al.* 2007). There is also a substantial literature suggesting that migration can fuel HIV; both by placing migrants themselves at greater risk of infection and because of the broader social turmoil it creates. Research has shown this to be the case in South Africa (see Abdool Karim *et al.* 1992; Lurie 2000; Zuma *et al.* 2003) and in other parts of Africa (Nunn *et al.* 1995; Lydie *et al.* 2004). Relevant to migration, as we shall see, there is also now a large amount of research in South Africa that shows how unemployment, poverty and sex/money exchanges can fuel multiple-sexual partners, sometimes across large age gaps (Hunter 2002; Selikow *et al.* 2002; LeClerc-Madlala 2003; for a review of the broader sub-Saharan literature, see Luke 2003). Women's movement is connected to these dynamics in much more complex ways than can be touched upon in this short chapter.

## Beyond the male migrant: a changing political economy of intimacy

Migrant labour, an institution entrenched in the nineteenth century after the discovery of gold and diamonds, restricted Africans from settling in urban areas and forced men into long absences from their rural homes. While the male-migrant-infector model was not the only social model used to understand the contemporary HIV pandemic in South Africa, it became one of the important ways in which the disease was framed, especially in the early years of the epidemic.

For sure, male migrancy was a central institution shaping households in twentieth-century South Africa. The country's geography became starkly divided by 'race' and most 'African' male workers were discouraged, often violently, from settling permanently in urban areas and instead forced back to languishing rural 'reserves', later called 'Bantustans'. Grossly unequal land distribution meant that rural areas for black South Africans shifted from a position where they subsidized low urban wages to a scenario where they depended on migrant men's remittances. However, from roughly the mid-1970s it is possible to tentatively trace a different constellation of forces shaping intimate relations; three interconnected social dimensions are particularly important to understand: (1) rising unemployment; (2) rapidly declining marital rates; and (3) the growth in women's movement/migration (I use the term 'movement' at times to emphasize how changes in location are often short term). I touch on points one and two only very briefly here and emphasize point three.[5] It is important to recognize that the rhythm and effects of all three of these changes are different. The mid-1970s signals the rise of chronic unemployment. However, reductions in marital rates started slightly earlier and women's migration probably increased in the late 1970s and certainly accelerated after the mid-1980s when apartheid's urban regulations totally collapsed.

### Unemployment and the changing household

Under apartheid, work for African men and women was typically dangerous, humiliating, and insecure. Nevertheless, because of high economic growth in the apartheid era (with steady growth after 1948 and accelerated growth in the 1960s) the labour of young African men and, to lesser extent women, was in heavy demand. All of this changed decisively from the mid-1970s as economic and political crisis shook the country. The first casualties of economic crisis were African men; a new class of men who had never been formally employed quickly came into existence. In the 1980s, women were drawn into factory work in increasing numbers but by the 1990s they were joining men in the ranks of the unemployed. From 1995 to 2005 unemployment rose by 12 per cent to 72 per cent for 15–24-year-old women and by 11 per cent to 58 per cent for men of the same age (Department of Labour 2006: 18).

In the post-apartheid period, many argue that market-led economic policy has accentuated social inequalities.[6] Seemingly shell-shocked by the perceived power of 'globalization', the government retreated from an interventionist economic and social strategy and embraced one that stressed growth through the market. Rapid trade liberalization, one element of this broadly neoliberal programme, dramatically increased wage competition and placed sectors such as clothing under great pressure, helping to nudge unemployment up to over 40 per cent (Nattrass 2003). As rural areas continued their decline, therefore, women were *pushed* into poorly remunerated and highly unstable informal work (Casale and Posel 2002); consequently, women's median income fell sharply in the post-apartheid period (Casale 2004). Added to these labour market changes was the AIDS pandemic itself that accentuated social inequalities, including gendered inequalities (Marais 2005). These forces drove a wedge between rich and poor and have not been adequately countered by state interventions such as increases to the value of the old age pension and the introduction of a child support grant aimed at assisting children up to the age of 15.

What is significant about the present generation of young South Africans, therefore, is that they are experiencing a simultaneous collapse of agrarian *and* wage livelihoods. This has very important consequences for marriage, household formation and sexuality. Marriage has always been a process and not an event and yet the task of building a household (denoted in *isiZulu* by the emotive metaphor *ukwakha umuzi*) is not achievable for many South Africans today in an era of chronic unemployment. According to the most recent population census, held in 2001, less than 30 per cent of African men and women over 15 years of age were in marital relations.[7] The factors behind this shift are complex; they include (until recently) women's increased work prospects and thus their growing economic independence from men. But particularly from the mid-1970s, when unemployment rose sharply, men's inability to secure *ilobolo* (bridewealth) or act as dependable 'providers' became additional brakes on marriage. Among many South Africans, wedlock is being exposed as a decidedly inflexible institution through which to organize social alliances and the flow of resources (cf. Niehaus 1994). Yet *ilobolo* is not fading in significance; rather, women typically see it as important precisely because it signifies men's commitment to them in an insecure world.

### Women's increased movement

Male migrant labour came to symbolize South Africa's racial structuring of society and overwhelms almost all discussions on migration. Yet for over a century southern African women have moved to towns, informal settlements, and white-owned farms (Bonner 1990; Walker 1990). The ending of influx controls (that sought to restrict Africans from entering towns) in 1986 is typically noted as the main driving force behind increases in women's recent movement and undoubtedly this is an important reason. But I want to suggest that this interacts with a relatively new set of dynamics: the reorganization of rural households into more geographically flexible institutions with an expectation that women as well as men will migrate, sometimes in circular patterns. The extent of these new patterns of movement has not adequately been captured by national statistics (although represented for some time in accounts by anthropologists, e.g. Spiegel 1995).

The census and annual household surveys (the latter conducted since 1993) are two key sources of national data on women's migration. Together, these show a rise in women's migration from the 1970s and, it appears, a particularly rapid rise in the 1990s (see Posel and Casale 2003; Kok *et al*. 2003; Posel 2006). Posel's (2006) analysis shows particularly well increases in women's movement in the 1990s; in 1993, an estimated 30 per cent of African migrant workers in South Africa were women but by only 1999 this had increased to approximately 34 per cent of migrant workers. She was also able to determine that in 1993 considerably more female migrants were unmarried then married (around 12 per cent compared with 3.5 per cent). The presence of an employed man in a household also deterred migration whereas the presence of a female pensioner seemed to facilitate migration. The latter is particularly important because pension payments have risen significantly after apartheid and enable a grandmother to care for her daughter's children. Taken together, these findings support the view that women's migration is connected to declines in marriage and the spatial reorganization of the household.

More intensively researched but geographically smaller demographic studies are able to provide important additional details. The Africa Centre for Population and Health Studies is based in Hlabisa, a mostly rural part of northern KwaZulu-Natal. It visits each household in a geographical area that it calls the Demographic Surveillance Areas every six months. It is therefore able to document in some detail the lives of the area's 85,000 strong population and better able than national data to capture shorter-term 'movements', a pattern more followed by women, especially those who leave children in rural areas (the census data, for instance, tend to capture movements over larger areas and for longer time spans). One notable finding is that there are now only slightly more women than men living in the rural area (around five per cent more). The study also found a steady rise in women's migration from 2000 and that gross migration rates (in and out migration taken together) were nearly the same for women as men (see Muhwava and Nyirenda 2007).[8]

Although there is undoubtedly great variety in women's movement patterns, what is clear is that most women no longer wait in rural areas to be infected by their migrant partners, the pattern of infection described convincingly in the 1940s for syphilis. We should remind ourselves that in the 1940s, the period when virtually all men were forced to move to urban areas to find work, rural areas were predominantly occupied on a day-to-day basis by children, women of all ages, and older men: one survey conducted by Kark (1950) in KwaZulu-Natal found that for peak ages of migrancy over *four times* as many men than women were absent from rural areas for more than one month of the year. Today, as noted, the difference in the number of men and women living in rural areas is small. It is also worth noting that in many cases today, rural-based women actually seem to infect their partners with HIV, and not the other way around. One study of discordant couples (where only one partner is infected) in rural KwaZulu-Natal showed that in 4 out of 10 cases it was actually women and not their partners who were HIV positive (Lurie *et al.* 2000), thus challenging the view that it is predominantly male migrants who infect their partners.

### Movement and new spaces

Although patterns of migration are extremely complex, one window into recent economic and demographic changes comes through the tremendous recent growth of informal settlements (sometimes called shack settlements). There is, to be sure, great variety in the constitution of these spaces. Informal settlements are typically seen as resulting from rural migrants streaming into large towns but this image tends to hide the fact that many residents hail from urban areas themselves. It also ignores the fact that informal settlements are a common feature of much smaller towns across South Africa (for insights into the many variations in informal settlements see Crankshaw 1993 and Huchzermeyer 2004).

What is important, and surprisingly rarely analyzed, is that informal settlements today appear to have nearly twice as high HIV prevalence than rural and urban areas (Human Science Research Council 2002, 2005). The earliest of these studies also found that urban informal areas contained the highest reported rates of multiple-partnered relationships (Human Science Research Council 2002). Of course, even if these figures are accurate (and we must maintain some scepticism) sexual practices can only partly explain such large geographical variations in HIV prevalence; higher infection rates in informal settlements compared with richer areas are in part a consequence of inadequate water, nutrition, and sanitation and the general poor state of health in the former.

But the high HIV prevalence rates in informal settlements certainly suggest taking a second look at connections between migration, marriage, the household, and the geographical manifestations of these institutions. One important feature of the late and post-apartheid period is the large 'unbundling' of households. Evidence of the proliferation of smaller, single, households is strong: from 1995 to 2002 average household size reduced from 4.3 to 3.8, driven by a rising share of single households from 12.6 per cent to 21 per cent of all households (Pirouz 2004). Indeed, despite the new government building over a million low-cost houses up to 2003 from 1996 to 2003 the number of informal dwellings, which are typically small households, rose by 688,000 (*Mail and Guardian* 2005).[9] Informal settlements today therefore are not only testimony to high unemployment rates and an inadequate government housing strategy but to significant demographic trends, namely the rise of smaller households not formed around a marital bond and the movement of both men and women.

My own ethnographic research brings these trends to bear on questions of HIV infection. This was mostly conducted at or near Isithebe Informal Settlement in the Mandeni municipality on the North Coast of the KwaZulu-Natal province. At the beginning of the twentieth century, the area was designated as 'tribal' land where only Africans could reside. In 1971, the apartheid state established Isithebe Industrial Park in the area as part of its strategy to reduce migration to large urban 'white' towns. It was on tribal land surrounding Isithebe's factories that Isithebe informal settlement grew (this is where the author stayed). In the 1990s, many scholars felt that the collapse of apartheid would herald a return to 'normal' migration patterns – settlement patterns would be concentrated around (rising) employment opportunities and migrants would not be forced to maintain such strong links with rural areas. But in the 1990s Isithebe informal settlement, like many others, continued to mushroom despite a decline in employment, in the Isithebe area from around 23,000 jobs in 1990 to roughly 15,000 by the end of the decade. What is more, movement rates continued to be high with migrants generally keeping a foothold in rural KwaZulu-Natal. Put simply many people who migrated to Isithebe in the 1990s did not find work and did not consider themselves permanent residents.

Women in Isithebe depend on a myriad of informal sector activities, from selling *dagga* (marijuana) to petty trading. But the sexual economy is also an increasingly important mechanism for the redistribution of formal and informal earnings and the provision of shelter for migrant women. That many migrant women do indeed have relationships with sometimes multiple men for money in the area is demonstrated by the commonly heard phrase 'one for rent, one for food, one for clothes' (see Hunter 2002). When considering this materiality of sex it is important to distinguish everyday intimate relations that involve sex/money exchanges from 'prostitution' – an activity that most residents say is rare in Isithebe. Most intimate relations, while widening women's ability to make claims on resources, are not simply instrumental: some partners can co-habit, gifts are often enacted in terms of men's 'provider' role, claims can be made through evoking 'love', and participants frequently discuss sexual pleasure and physical attraction.[10] It is common to hear stories of women having relationships linked to material gifts but also common to hear about love letters and signs of affection. A final important point to recognize is that these sexual networks operate alongside – and not in opposition to – social networks based on kinship, friendship groups, churches, and neighbours.

In many cases therefore, sex exchanges do not cause family breakdown, a fact that questions the very long association between 'prostitution' and 'social degeneration'. On the contrary, remittances from sexual networks can help to foster kinship ties. There is an expectation that women will furnish money to a rural home, especially if a woman's child is looked after by other family members. Earlier scholarship showed how men's urban wages were distributed through sexual networks in rural Lesotho (Spiegel 1981) and how rigid conjugal bonds in South Africa were being superseded by more flexible *sibling* bonds characterized by reciprocity (Niehaus 1994). What is different today is how women's migration further reflects and affects this changing household structure. In a situation where marital bonds are no longer common, one model is where rural women can pivot multiple movements around their rural home (sometimes where a child is left), a fairly flexible arrangement allowing for women's frequent movement, the transfer of resources through sexual liaisons, and the redistribution of state benefits, especially pensions, often through the presence of a rural grandparent, usually a *gogo* (granny). As unemployment bites deeper into society, sexual exchanges and the household have been interwoven in new ways.

## Conclusions

In the last decade, political economists have rightly stressed how the social roots of South Africa's AIDS pandemic lie in apartheid. Yet in the early period of AIDS male migration tended to be projected forward to explain current circumstances. Although the model's appeal waned over time, it contributed to policy makers overlooking the *interconnected* economic, spatial, and demographic landscape today that are so vital to the continued unfolding of the South African AIDS pandemic. Of course, migration is a messy process and difficult to capture. And the patterns described here are by no means comprehensive. Yet important to any understanding must be recognition of radical recent changes to the political economy and geography of intimacy, particularly the sharp decline in marital rates and the rise of unemployment. These interacted with shifts in masculinities, femininities, and indeed the very idea of the 'family', 'love', and 'sex' in ways that this chapter has not considered (see for instance, in relation to KwaZulu-Natal, Hunter 2005). These connections and others must be more fully teased out and emphasized if prevention campaigns are to resonate with the social conditions in which many South Africans, and indeed other groups, live.

## Notes

1 Under colonialism and apartheid, South Africans were divided into distinct 'racial' groups. By the end of the apartheid era there were four categories that are still widely used today: African, White, Indian, and Coloured. Although clearly problematic, without using these terms it is very difficult to understand the processes through which race can structure, and be structured by, society and space. I use scare quotes conservatively to improve this article's readability.

2 This chapter is based on ethnographic research conducted in Mandeni, KwaZulu-Natal, where I lived extensively with a family in Isithebe Informal Settlement between 2000 and 2006, and on secondary and archival research. I am unable to give extensive background to the study because of space limitations, but see Hunter (2002, 2005).

3 For an excellent recent history of same-sex relationships in southern Africa see Epprecht (2004). On connections between sexual violence and HIV prevalence see Dunkle *et al.* (2004).

4 These figures are taken from annual studies conducted at antenatal sites. See Marais (2005: 25–43) for a thorough discussion of South African AIDS statistics.

5 A fuller version of some of the themes described here can be found at Hunter (2007). This chapter draws extensively, in parts, on this article.

6 See Seekings and Nattrass (2005). On neo-liberalism in post-apartheid South Africa see Marais (2001).

7 According to census figures, the number of married African people above 15 years was as follows: 1936 – 56 per cent; 1951 – 54 per cent; 1960 – 57 per cent; 1970 – 49 per cent; 1980 – 42 per cent; 1991 – 38 per cent; 2001 – 30 per cent (author's calculation from various census reports, Statistics South Africa, Pretoria). The age of 15 is arbitrarily chosen but commonly used in census data on marriage. Notably, marital rates appear to have fallen much faster in South Africa than in other parts of the region; see Hosegood and Preston-Whyte (2002) for figures on Botswana, Namibia, and Zimbabwe.

8 A demographic surveillance site in northern east South Africa (Agincourt) also found an increasing mobility of women, although it appears at a lesser scale than that recorded in Hlabisa (differences in the way the surveys are constructed make comparisons difficult). See Kok and Collinson (2006).

9 By 2008, the government had built 2 million houses and yet informal settlements were still prominent.

10 For an excellent discussion of gift exchanges and intimacy in Brazil, see Rebhun (1999). The nature of these relationships is important: while policy makers tend to see low condom use in narrow terms of 'male power', it is often in affairs between 'boyfriends' and 'girlfriends' – positioned as being about love – where men and women are least likely to use condoms and in the most commodified relationships, prostitution, where condoms are used the most (e.g. Smith 2004).

## References

Abdool Karim, Q., Abdool Karim, S., Singh, B., Short, R., and Ngxongo, S. (1992) 'Seroprevalence of HIV infection in rural South Africa', *AIDS*, 6: 1535–39.

Bonner, P. (1990) 'Desirable or undesirable Basotho women? Liquor, prostitution and the migration of Basotho women to the Rand, 1920–45', in C. Walker (ed.), *Women and Gender in Southern Africa to 1945*, Cape Town: David Philip.

Casale, D. (2004) 'What has the feminisation of the labour market bought women in South Africa? Trends in labour force participation, employment and earnings', 1995–2001. *Development Policy Research Unit (Cape Town) Working Paper, 04.*

Casale, D. and Posel, D., (2002) 'The continued feminisation of the labour force in South Africa: an analysis of recent data and trends', *The South African Journal of Economics*, 70(1): 168–95.

Crankshaw, O. (1993) 'Squatting, apartheid, and urbanisation on the southern Witwatersrand', *African Affairs*, 92(366): 31–51.

Department of Labour (2006) *Women in the South African Labour Market*, Pretoria: Department of Labour.

Dunkle, K. L., Jewkes, R. K., Brown, H. C., Gray, G. E., McIntryre, J. A., and Harlow, S. D. (2004) 'Gender-based violence, relationship power, and risk of HIV infection in women attending antenatal clinics in South Africa', *Lancet*, 363(9419): 1415–21.

Epprecht, M. (2004) *Hungochani: The History of a Dissident Sexuality in Southern Africa*, Montréal, QC: McGill-Queen's University Press.

Farmer, P. (1999) *Infections and Inequalities: The Modern Plagues*, Berkeley, California: University of California Press.

Hirsch, J. S. and Wardlow, H. (2006) *Modern Loves: The Anthropology of Romantic Courtship and Companionate Marriage*, Ann Arbor, Michigan: University of Michigan Press.

Hosegood, V. and Preston-Whyte, E. (2002) 'Marriage and partnership patterns in rural KwaZulu Natal, South Africa', session 33. Social consequences of AIDS, Population Association of America, 8–12 May, Atlanta.

Huchzermeyer, M. (2004) *Unlawful Occupation: Informal Settlements and Urban Policy in South Africa and Brazil*, Trenton, New Jersey: Africa World Press.

Human Science Research Council (2002) *Nelson Mandela/HSRC Study of AIDS*, Cape Town: HSRC.

——(2005) *South African National HIV Prevalence, HIV Incidence, Behaviour and Communication Survey*, Cape Town: HSRC Press.

Hunter, M. (2002) 'The materiality of everyday sex: thinking beyond "prostitution"', *African Studies*, 61(1): 99–120.

——(2005) 'Cultural politics and masculinities: multiple-partners in historical perspective in KwaZulu-Natal', *Culture, Health, and Sexuality*, 7(4): 389–403.

——(2007) 'The changing political economy of sex in South Africa: the significance of unemployment and inequalities to the scale of the AIDS pandemic', *Social Science & Medicine*, 64(3): 689–700.

Kark, S. (1949) 'The social pathology of syphilis in Africans', *South African Medical Journal*, 23, 77–84.

——(1950) 'The influence of urban–rural migration on Bantu Health and Disease', *The Leech*, 23–37.

Kok, P. and Collinson, M. (2006) 'Migration and urbanization in South Africa', report 03.04.02, Pretoria: Statistics South Africa.

Kok, P., O'Donovan, M., Bouare, O., and Van Zyl, J. (2003) *Post-apartheid Patterns of Internal Migration in South Africa*, Pretoria: Human Science Research Council.

LeClerc-Madlala, S. (2003) 'Transactional sex and the pursuit of modernity', *Social Dynamics*, 29(2): 213–33.

Luke, N. (2003) 'Age and economic asymmetries in the sexual relationships of adolescent girls in sub-Saharan Africa', *Studies in Family Planning*, 34(2): 67–86.

Lurie, M. (2000) 'Migration and AIDS in Southern Africa: a review', *South African Journal of Science*, 96: 343–47.

Lurie, M., Williams, B., Zuma, K., Mkaya-Mwamburi, D., Garnett, G., and Sweat, M. *et al.* (2000) 'Who infects whom? HIV-1 concordance and discordance among migrants and non-migrant couples in South Africa', *AIDS*, 17: 2245–52.

Lydie, N., Robinson, N., Ferry, B., Akam, E., De Loenzien, M., and Abega, S. (2004) 'Mobility, sexual behavior, and HIV infection in an urban population in Cameroon', *Journal of Acquired Immune Deficiency Syndrome*, 35(1): 67–74.

*Mail and Guardian.* (2005) 'The rise and rise of South Africa's shacks', January 6, 2006.

Marais, H. (2001) *South Africa, Limits to Change: The Political Economy of Transformation*, London: Zed.

——(2005) *Buckling. The Impact of AIDS in South Africa*, Pretoria: University of Pretoria.

McClintock, A. (1995) *Imperial Leather: Race, Gender, and Sexuality in the Colonial Conquest*, New York; London: Routledge.

Muhwava, W. and Nyirenda, M. (2007) 'Demographic and socio-economic trends in the ACDIS', Monograph No 2, Africa Centre for Health and Population Studies, Mtubatuba, South Africa.

Nattrass, N. (2003) 'The state of the economy: a crisis of employment', in J. Daniel, A. Habib and R. Southall (eds), *State of the Nation. South Africa 2003–4*, Cape Town: HSRC Press.

Niehaus, I. (1994) 'Disharmonious spouses and harmonious siblings: conceptualising household formation among urban residents in QwaQwa', *African Studies*, 53(1): 115–35.

Nunn, A., Wagner, H., Kamali, A., Kengeya-Kayondo, J., and Mulder, D. (1995) 'Migration and HIV-1 seroprevalence in a rural Ugandan population', *AIDS*, 9: 503–6.

Padilla, M. B., Hirsch, J. S., Munoz-Laboy, M., Sember, R., and Parker, R. (2007) *Love and Globalization: Transformations of Intimacy in the Contemporary World*, Nashville, Tennessee: Vanderbilt University Press.

Pirouz, F. (2004) 'Have labour market outcomes affected household structure in South Africa? A preliminary descriptive analysis of households', Paper for Conference on African Development and Poverty Reduction, Cape Town, October 13–15.

Posel, D. (2006) 'Moving on: patterns of labour migration in post-apartheid South Africa', in M. Tienda, S. Findley, S. Tollman, E. Preston-Whyte (eds), *Africa on the Move*, Johannesburg: Witwatersrand University Press.

Posel, D. and Casale, D. (2003) 'What has been happening to internal labour migration in South Africa, 1993–99?' *The South African Journal of Economics*, 71(3): 455–79.

Rebhun, L. (1999) *The Heart is Unknown Country: Love in the Changing Economy of Northeast Brazil*, Stanford, California: Stanford University Press.

Schoepf, B., Schoepf, C., and Millen, J. (2000) 'Theoretical therapies, remote remedies: SAPs and the political ecology of poverty and health in Africa', in *Dying for Growth. Global Inequality and the Health of the Poor*, Monroe, Maine: Common Courage Press.

Seekings, J. and Nattrass, N. (2005) *Class, Race, and Inequality in South Africa*, New Haven: Yale University Press.

Selikow, T., Zulu, B., and Cedras, E. (2002) 'The ingagara, the regte and the cherry. HIV/AIDS and youth culture in contemporary urban townships', *Agenda*, 53: 22–32.

Smith, D. (2004) 'Premarital sex, procreation and HIV risk in Nigeria', *Studies in Family Planning*, 35(4): 223–35.

Spiegel, A. (1981) 'Changing patterns of migrant labour and rural differentiation in Lesotho', *Social Dynamics*, 6(2): 1–13.

——(1995) 'Migration, urbanisation and domestic fluidity: reviewing some South African examples', *African Anthropology*, II(2): 90–113.

Stillwaggon, E. (2006) *AIDS and the Ecology of Poverty*, Oxford; New York: Oxford University Press.

Vaughan, M. (1991) *Curing Their Ills: Colonial Power and African Illness*, Stanford, California: Stanford University Press.

Walker, C. (1990) 'Gender and the development of the migrant labour system c. 1850–1930: An overview', in C. Walker (ed.), *Women and Gender in Southern Africa to 1945*, Cape Town: David Philip.

Zuma, K., Gouws, E., Williams, B., and Lurie, M. (2003) 'Risk factors for HIV infection among women in Carletonville, South Africa: Migration, demography and sexually transmitted diseases', *International Journal of STD & AIDS*, 14: 814–17.

# Chapter 12

# Labour migration and risky sexual behaviour

## Tea plantation workers in Kericho District, Kenya

*Kennedy Nyabuti Ondimu*

Studies of migration in a number of developing countries have found that people who are mobile are often likely to be at higher risk of HIV infection than those who do not move, largely because mobility may be associated with risky sexual behaviours (Lurie *et al.* 2003; Ondimu 2005; UN 2005; Chinaglia *et al.* 2008). Several factors have been proposed to explain the link between mobility and sexual risk, such as the fact that people tend to migrate at ages when they are most sexually active (UN 2005), separation of couples and demand for commercial sex (Pison *et al.* 1993), cultural changes (Decosas *et al.* 1995), socio-economic and living conditions (Flournoy and Yen 2004; Hallman 2004), and modifications of gender-based power relations (Gupta and Weiss 1993; Mason 1994; Fapohunda and Rutenberg 1999; Blanc 2001).

This chapter addresses some of the above, with a special emphasis on gender norms, the widespread patterns of behaviour that are generally tolerated or accepted as proper, reinforced by others, and sometimes quite hard for individuals to resist (Tibandebage and Mackintosh 2002). After describing the living and working conditions of migrant workers on tea plantations in the Kericho district of Kenya, I discuss the workers' HIV-related knowledge and behaviours. I show how sexual risk takes place as a function of factors operating at individual, household and community levels, and how gender imbalances influence migration to work away from one's home community, living and working conditions at destination, and sexual risk behaviours.

The chapter is based on findings from a study in which, following preliminary focus group discussions, a household survey was carried out amongst a random 10 per cent sample of male and female workers on six of Kericho's 27 tea estates. A standard Knowledge, Attitudes, Practices and Beliefs questionnaire was administered in face-to-face interviews with a total of 630 workers. In a third phase of the study sexual and sexually transmitted infection/HIV-related behaviour, perceptions, and experiences were explored in 60 in-depth interviews with a broad range of sexually active workers. The interview format in this phase allowed extensive rapport to build, permitting exploration of complex, ambiguous and potentially sensitive material (Ondimu 2005).

## Tea production and plantation workers in Kericho

Tea farming was brought to Kenya from India by European settler farmers as early as 1903, making Kenya the oldest tea producer in Africa, and the world's largest tea exporter today. Kenyan tea is grown mainly in the highlands east and west of the rift valley, where the tropical climate and rich volcanic soils give it unique flavour and character. The beverage is produced both on small 0.2 to 12 hectare farms and on large plantations averaging 700 hectares, owned by multinational corporations or by private individuals. A typical tea plantation, made up of self-contained farms and a tea processing factory, employs over 10,000 workers, all of whom live at the estate. Tea plantations are among the largest providers of wage employment in Kenya. The Kericho district contains a large proportion of the country's tea farms, employing some 35,000 workers in 2002 (Republic of Kenya 2003) and making the district a major destination for semi-skilled labour migration from the densely populated neighbouring Nyanza and Western provinces in the Lake Victoria Basin.

Tea production is labour-intensive, especially during picking and transportation. Two leaves and the bud are manually plucked from bushes, placed in a basket usually carried on the picker's back, then carried to a factory for processing. Figure 12.1 shows tea pickers at work Kericho.

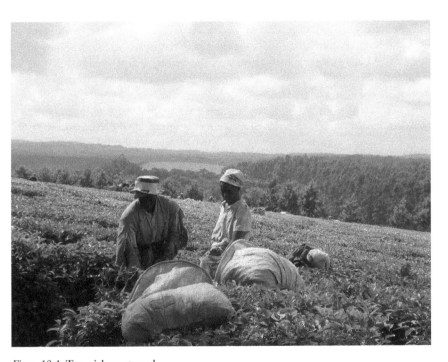

*Figure 12.1* Tea pickers at work

Although picking tea was initially considered a 'man's job' because of the physical demands of the work, over 30 per cent of tea plantation workers are currently women (Ondimu 2005). Men who move to Kericho in search of employment are mainly either young unmarried men who have left school early, or married men who migrate alone in hopes of finding employment that will allow them to send remittances home to their families. A small third group of male tea workers has migrated from rural regions to escape community wrath after having been involved in criminal activities. Whatever the category, male migrants are likely to move alone, leaving any wives and children at home.

Female labour migrants, on the other hand, are likely to have migrated to Kericho with dependants. A small proportion of them are married to male tea workers. Most, however, are separated, divorced, or unmarried mothers with children. One of the factors pushing women to migrate is the patriarchal nature of their rural communities of origin. In the Kisii, Luo, and Luhya communities from which the majority originates, men own the land, and women have no right to inherit or to own property. Women are absorbed into their husband's family at marriage, and a culture of son preference reigns. Girls are widely discriminated against in access to education: expected to combine school attendance with domestic labour, girls' performance at school is poor, and they drop out early. The practice of bride price is still common, and pushes some parents to force their daughters to marry early. When marriages break up, daughters return to their natal homes, but they are received with hostility. Women from broken marriages are thus denied access to resources of their own, and – restricted in their ability to provide for their now 'fatherless' children – they have little choice but to migrate to find work in the nearby tea plantations.

Some of the characteristics of the tea plantation workers surveyed in 2004 are presented in Table 12.1.

In the present study, most of the workers migrated from rural areas, typically from traditional village societies. The largest proportion, the Kisii, come from the densely populated neighbouring districts, followed by the Luo, Kalenjin and Luhya. While almost all had attended some school, the majority left after the primary level. On average, female workers spent fewer years in school than their male counterparts. The low levels of education are reflected in plantation workers' ability to read and write: one-third of the men and half of the women have difficulty reading, or are unable to do so. Processing tea is the only source of income for most. Four men and three women out of 10 said they had never been married, whereas higher proportions of women than men said they were separated, divorced or widowed.

As for living conditions, plantation management provides housing for tea workers. Little alternative is available since a lack of commercial land in adjacent areas prevents development of private for-rent houses. Originally meant for single male occupants, most of the estate housing units have shared toilets, bathrooms and kitchens. Most do not have electricity. There are few adequate recreational and religious facilities on the residential estates, and only a small

*Table 12.1* Kericho tea plantation workers: selected characteristics 2004 (in %, n=630)

|  | Males (n=450) | Females (n=180) |
|---|---|---|
| *Age (average)* | 28.2 | 22.4 |
| *Former residence* | | |
| Rural | 68.9 | 84.4 |
| Urban | 31.1 | 15.6 |
| *Ethnic group* | | |
| Kisi | 41.1 | 31.7 |
| Kalenjin | 16.0 | 15.0 |
| Luo | 24.0 | 28.9 |
| Luhya | 8.9 | 7.2 |
| Kikuyu | 10.0 | 12.2 |
| Other | 1.1 | 2.2 |
| *Level of schooling attained* | | |
| None | 1.8 | 6.7 |
| Pre-primary | 0.9 | 4.4 |
| Primary | 67.8 | 71.7 |
| Secondary and above | 29.6 | 17.2 |
| *Ability to read* | | |
| Not at all | 14.7 | 24.4 |
| With difficulty | 18.9 | 28.3 |
| Easily | 64.4 | 47.2 |
| *Other source of income available* | | |
| None | 78.0 | 82.2 |
| Business | 2.2 | 6.1 |
| Spouse/partner's employment | 6.0 | 4.4 |
| Other | 13.8 | 7.2 |
| *Current marital status* | | |
| Single/never married | 38.0 | 30 |
| Separated | 14.9 | 24.4 |
| Widowed | 1.1 | 6.7 |
| Divorced | 2.2 | 8.3 |
| Married/cohabiting | 43.8 | 30.6 |

number of workers go to church. Most female workers spend their free time with their children, or doing housework, knitting, making baskets or mending. Male workers play football, and a few engage in petty trading or work on vegetable gardens. Figure 12.2 shows one of the residential camps in the tea plantations, with units close to each other and communal pit latrines next to the blocks.

Housing conditions have not kept pace with increases in labour force or with changes in household demographics, in particular with the fact that most workers now live with large families: the average household currently contains four to eight persons, and most dwellings accommodate more than one household. In addition, people from different tribes, religions and geographical areas live

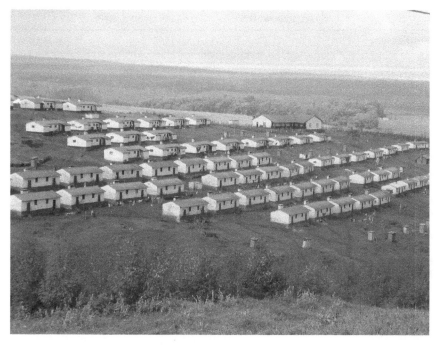

*Figure 12.2* Workers residential estate in Kericho

together in circumstances under which traditional cultural beliefs and norms may not operate, and nuclear families are away from the support of the extended family. Migrant women, in particular, are left to cope on their own: their relatives are unlikely to be available to help with child care as they would in the communities of origin, and neighbours from different areas, traditions and ethnic groups are not likely to be willing to give support. Although intermarriages between the different groups are now common, a community of such ethnic diversity rarely provides the level of support needed in times of stress, illness or unemployment. Instead, diversity leads to tension, community violence and insecurity. Violence and insecurity are fed by inadequate security coverage in the area, social exclusion, and drug and alcohol dependency. The main victims of sexual and domestic violence are unmarried women workers and children: single women and those in female-headed households report being the object of insults, harassment and abuse from males, both at work and at home. Indeed, exposure to stress, harassment and abuse was cited as a reason for female workers to seek protection from male partners, sometimes in return for sexual favours.

In sum, living conditions in the tea estates are comparable to those found in urban slums, with small overcrowded dwellings, limited access to water and inadequate sanitation, and lack of electricity. In in-depth interviews conducted as part of the study, workers described their residential areas as noisy and crowded, offering little privacy. The lack of recreational activities creates idleness for male workers, especially, leaving them available for excessive drinking of the cheap brew that is sold clandestinely. Conditions are thus ideal for physical and sexual violence, as well as contributing to risky sexual behaviour. As one man put it:

> How can you talk about counselling people on safe sex when a single man lives in the same compound and shares a toilet, bathroom with a single lady who is willing to sell sex? The temptations will be always there!
>
> (cited in Ondimu 2005: 88)

## Employment and working conditions

Most tea plantation workers are hired as temporary casual labourers, and paid only for the days actually worked. Monthly wages are determined mainly by the amount of tea picked, which depends on the number of hours worked and the weather conditions, as well as on the worker's skill and physical fitness. Absence from work, for whatever reason, means no money for that time, and frequent absenteeism can result in dismissal. A few experienced tea plantation workers are engaged on permanent terms, although they are expected to pick a certain amount of tea per day, and paid less if they fail to meet the quota. Permanent workers are entitled to annual leaves to travel to visit their rural families, but since they receive no salary during this time most opt not to take the leave. Only a small proportion belongs to the Kenya Plantation Workers' Union. Medical care is covered by the employer, but dependants' medical expenses must be met by the workers themselves.

Men work for an average of 10 hours per day, seven days a week, whereas women, with their additional domestic and child care responsibilities, work an average of eight hours, and six days a week. Since monthly payments depend on the weight of the tea picked, female workers end up earning significantly less than their male counterparts: average monthly income for men was just under 6,000 Kenyan Shillings at the time the study was carried out, whereas it was 3,605 for women (approximately 84 and 51 US dollars, respectively). Unlike in rural areas, where people can survive for periods of time without money, life in the tea plantations depends on cash for such essentials as clothing, food, medical care, and children's schooling. Since the majority of tea plantation workers have no other sources of income, and since they usually have no reserves, loss of income means immediate loss of food. Several other factors also affect food security and nutrition, including loss of the small plots of land formerly provided for subsistence gardens; the fact that female heads of household are unable to rely on food support from their rural families as male workers do; and the long working hours which, apart from leaving workers little time to cultivate or to search for food, mean that workers have no lunch break and that children are left to fend for themselves at noon or to eat something prepared for them before their mothers leave for work.

Although working conditions in the tea plantations are poor, workers have few other employment opportunities and turnover rates are low. Mobility for female workers, in particular, is restricted by the low levels of schooling, family obligations, and hostile conditions at home just discussed. Most female workers never return to their rural homes: they are likely to change status only if they marry and move to live with their husbands.

## HIV knowledge and awareness

The past several years have seen a marked increase in HIV-related deaths in Kenya's tea plantations (Liyala *et al.* 2000). In a study conducted in 2006, HIV-1 prevalence among Kericho tea plantations residents was 14.3 per cent, considerably higher than the national average of six per cent, and higher among women (19.1 per cent) than among men (11.3 per cent) (Foglia *et al.* 2007). An earlier study in the same area had shown prevalence for women as more than twice that of men (Sateren *et al.* 2006).

The government of Kenya, in collaboration with tea plantation managements, has carried out a range of HIV prevention programmes for plantation workers, including mass media health communication, peer education, prevention of mother-to-child transmission, and HIV treatment through anti-retroviral therapy. Significant efforts have been made to offer voluntary HIV counselling and testing (VCT) for workers, and several free VCT and heath care facilities are available. One of the aims of the present study was to assess the impact of such programmes – and help orient future programmes – by measuring workers' AIDS-related knowledge, perceptions, and behaviours.

Male and female workers' knowledge of HIV and AIDS was found to be generally good (see Ondimu 2005 for details). Almost everyone had heard about HIV and AIDS, and knew where to find condoms. Just over half of the respondents said they knew someone affected. A significant proportion had misconceptions, however: in particular one-quarter of the women denied knowing about maternal-to-child transmission. Only roughly half of the workers thought they themselves could be at risk of infection. Knowledge of VCT services was almost universal, but did not translate into utilization: only 10 per cent of male and 30 per cent of female workers said they had ever been tested for HIV, and only 27 per cent of the men and 52 per cent of the women said they would like to be. The reasons for non-utilization of VCT services were explored in the interviews: by far the main reason was heavy workload and inadequate free time, followed by absence of any symptoms. Most interviewees believed that a person with HIV or AIDS has clearly identifiable symptoms, and that the absence of such symptoms is a clear indication that one is 'clean': VCT is perceived to be for helping those already infected. One 25-year-old man explained it this way:

A tea picker's salary depends on the amount of tea leaves he picks per month. This work is physically demanding and to earn a salary of 3000 shillings per a month, you need to work over 10 hours a day for six days in a week. Unless one is very sick, we do not have spare time to visit a VCT for mere advice.

(cited in Ondimu 2005: 91)

The third major reason for avoiding HIV testing is the fear and confusion that may arise if one turns out to be infected. Discussants told stories about people who died within weeks of learning about their positive HIV status, and about people who committed suicide or took out bank loans to spend recklessly after a positive test. Other themes included fear of being stigmatized, and also that one might be deliberately infected with HIV during testing.

## Sexual behaviour

Both the survey and the in-depth interviews enquired about sexual behaviour. Table 12.2 presents selected results from the survey. Overall, only a small minority of the respondents reported currently having no sexual partner, and about one-third reported having a regular sexual partner. Two-thirds of the men and just over half of the women reported having occasional partners.

Seventy-eight per cent of the men reported having had penetrative sex with a person to whom they were not married in the month preceding the survey, as did 42 per cent of the women. Amongst these, 65 per cent of the men and 25 per cent of the woman said they had been under the influence of alcohol at the time. Forty per cent of the men and 22 per cent of the women responded yes to the questionnaire item asking if they had ever engaged in transactional sex. Factors influencing transactional sex were explored in the in-depth interviews. Shown in Table 12.3, these reflect the family separations, changes in social environment, social isolation, and sense of anonymity found among the tea plantation workers (Ondimu 2005) as well as the gender inequality already discussed.

*Table 12.2* Sexual behaviour among male and female workers (%, n=630)

| Risk behaviours | Males (n=450) | Females (n=180) |
|---|---|---|
| *Sexual partner* | | |
| Regular | 31.5 | 35.0 |
| Occasional | 64.9 | 52.8 |
| No partner | 3.6 | 12.2 |
| Extra marital sex in the previous month | 77.8 | 41.6 |
| Extramarital sex while drunk | 65.4 | 25.0 |
| Ever engaged in sex-for-cash | 40.0 | 22.0 |
| Non-use of condom during extramarital sex | 50.6 | 33.3 |

*Table 12.3* Factors responsible for extramarital sex: male and female tea workers (interview data)

| Males | | Females | |
|---|---|---|---|
| Reason | % citing | Reason | % citing |
| Need to satisfy sexual desire | 97 | Need for economic/financial assistance from males | 93 |
| Separation from wife/spouse | 90 | False promise of marriage | 92 |
| Men must have many sexual partners | 90 | Need for protection from a male partner | 90 |
| Availability of sex workers | 80 | Availability of men | 77 |
| Influence of alcohol | 67 | Influence of alcohol | 57 |
| Temptations high because of residential arrangements | 53 | There is nothing wrong with having many partners | 43 |
| Doesn't know that it's risky | 38 | | |

The motivations most commonly cited by male workers were the need to satisfy sexual desire, the belief that real men must have many sexual partners, the availability of sex workers in the urban areas adjacent to the tea plantations, and 'the tempting social environment' within the tea estates. Married men living away from their spouses explained that since it was not possible to support a large family within the estates, and that they sent money back to their families, their extramarital sex was justified by their situation, and necessary to satisfy their sexual needs. Interviewees also remarked that most male workers end up never making remittances to their rural homes, instead spending their earnings on beer, leisure and transactional sex. As for the increasing numbers of young unmarried workers the plantations are seeing, who have no strong attachment with their rural homes and who spend most of their earnings where they are currently living, interviewees noted that having a girlfriend gives prestige. Casual relations are supported by community beliefs that 'regular sex is necessary for good health' and 'men are by nature polygamous'. The men interviewed said the availability of sex workers in the nearby urban centres was a reason for male infidelity, noting that sex workers come to actively solicit male clients at the labour camps, bars and other places they congregate on paydays. Alcohol is also liberally consumed on paydays, with intoxication promoting increased sexual risk, especially with non-regular partners (Ondimu 2005).

Female workers cited quite different reasons for engaging in extramarital sex. Almost all said the main reason was for economic support from a man: female plantation workers are likely to be the sole source of support for their dependents, and poverty may drive them to engage in sex with casual partners in exchange for necessary basic resources. Somewhat similarly, female interviewees also frequently mentioned insecurity and the need for social and physical protection: many women feel they need to have a man around to protect them from high levels of physical violence and of bullying by male workers. Female discussants also cited a partner's false promise of marriage or re-marriage as a reason for engaging in sex. They explained that anyone not married by a certain age risks being seen as a social misfit, thus that unmarried women are vulnerable to being taken advantage of by men making promises they have no intention of fulfilling. Other themes commonly cited by female respondents included the availability of 'rich' men willing to buy sex, the influence of alcohol, and the idea that, after all, there is nothing wrong with having many sexual partners.

As shown in Table 12.2, only half the men and one-third of the women said they had used a condom during extramarital sex. This low use of condoms, combined with high HIV prevalence, implies high risks of exposure to infection, and is particularly striking in light of the high levels of HIV knowledge just described. The in-depth interviews help explain some of the influences at work: almost all of the male discussants felt that condoms interrupt sexual activity, cause discomfort and ruin the excitement, or that using them is a sign of weakness. Many also said that using condoms with their regular sexual partners would imply mistrust. Others were sceptical about the effectiveness of condoms, saying they tend to break during intercourse, that they may cause injuries, or even that condoms contain substances that can infect users. Female respondents gave different reasons for not using condoms with non-marital partners, many of which reflect their economically disadvantaged position, and also the norms that make negotiation difficult or impossible for women. Most said they do not use condoms simply because 'men don't like it', but 9 out of 10 also said a man might abandon a women who asked her partner to use a condom, and three-quarters said someone who did so might be construed as a prostitute or a woman of loose morals. Another important reason for women not using condoms, as for men, was mutual trust with the partner: one might use a condom for a first-time affair, but the need diminishes as the relationship develops. Many felt that a sexually transmitted infection such as gonorrhoea would serve as an indicator: if a person is not infected after an initial sexual contact then trust and commitment can increase. With a more regular partner condoms might be used to prevent pregnancy, but not for disease prevention. One male respondent put it this way:

> I have had sexual contact with this woman twice and I have not got any infection, even though we are not married. I trust her and do not see why I should use a condom. A condom is meant to protect pregnancy and my partner uses tablets (pills) which are more reliable.
>
> (cited in Ondimu 2005: 93)

## Concluding remarks

This study shows relatively high levels of HIV knowledge among tea plantation workers in Kenya. Almost all had heard about AIDS, and were aware that HIV can be transmitted through sexual intercourse. However, and although HIV prevalence on the plantations has been shown to be relatively high, a large proportion of workers still perceive themselves to be at low risk of infection. Seventy-eight per cent of the male workers and 42 per cent of the female workers said they had engaged in sexual relations with partner to whom they were not married in the previous month, and for more than half of the males and one-third of the females these contacts were unprotected by condoms. Numerous HIV testing and counselling services are available, but only a small proportion of tea plantation workers had used them. This risky behaviour places plantation workers at risk of infection, as it does their rural spouses, to whom male workers, especially, occasionally return for visits.

Several factors operating at community, household and individual levels, increase risky sexual behaviours for migrant workers. Community factors include perceptions of HIV and AIDS, the availability of commercial sex and the price of safe sex, and access to and use of heath services (Careal et al. 1994; Philipson and Posner 1995; Ahlburg et al. 1997; Ondimu 2005; Sen and Ostlin 2007). Tea estate communities were found to be marked by extreme economic deprivation and gender inequality, as well as by breakdown of community-induced migration: the support and guidance of the traditional extended family has disappeared, and nuclear families are left to cope with violence and drug and alcohol abuse.

At household level, most workers within the tea plantations live in crowded and unhygienic conditions, in precarious economic circumstances. Members of households in which one or more members abuse alcohol, and those with many dependants but few wage earners, were at especially high risk. Female-headed households were particularly vulnerable, because of large family size, the meagre income of the head of household (who in most cases is the sole breadwinner) and lack of food support from their rural extended families, a safety valve available to most male-headed households. Since households depend on cash for the purchase of essential goods low income increases the likelihood that women will engage in transactional sex to survive.

Several individual-level variables contribute to HIV-related sexual risk. For male workers these include being currently unmarried or separated from their wives and families, and community norms that promote the idea that a man must have many sex partners. For female workers, and apart from the needs for protection and to engage in 'survival sex' just mentioned, these include gender norms that decrease women's ability to engage in sex safely and on their own terms. For both sexes, low levels of schooling make it difficult for workers to find better paying jobs elsewhere – they have little alternative but to remain casual workers.

The findings suggest that a comprehensive set of measures is urgently needed to prevent the rapid growth of the HIV epidemic in the tea plantation sector in Kenya. A comprehensive HIV prevention programme is necessary, one that will take into account that over 40 per cent of the target population cannot use print media. The use of condoms must be promoted, and workers should be encouraged to assert their rights to resist unprotected sex. Routine voluntary HIV counselling and testing must be encouraged, and information must be given to combat incorrect ideas about VCT. A multifaceted HIV and AIDS workplace programme must be established, with a legal framework that will protect employees' rights, and protect them from stigma and discrimination, in particular from the fear that they will lose their jobs if they test HIV positive. An International Labour Organisation (ILO) code of practice on HIV and AIDS sets good standards in this respect (ILO 2001). Efforts must be made to empower women on tea plantations, by addressing norms that disadvantage females (Sen and Ostlin 2007; Chinaglia *et al.* 2008) and by removing imbalances in income levels that promote commercial sex. One way may be to help female workers start income-generating activities to diversify their sources of income. There is a need to improve housing conditions, and – once housing conditions improve – to encourage workers to migrate to the workplace with their spouses and families. Sports, educational and other leisure centres must be established. Closure of places that sell illicit liquor should be facilitated, and programmes established to reduce drug and alcohol abuse among plantation workers. Physical security must be increased, and there may be value in promoting religious activities, since there is evidence that high levels of religiosity are associated with key demographic and health outcomes (Smith 2003; Lehrer 2004; McQuillan 2004), lower the probability of substance abuse and antisocial behaviour among young people, and delay sexual debut and entry into cohabitation (Lehrer 2004).

In sum, while messages urging change in sexual behaviour are necessary, these alone are unlikely to yield substantial successes. Reducing HIV risk and vulnerability among tea plantation workers will require improving their working conditions, their economic welfare and their community conditions.

## Acknowledgement

This chapter is based on research funded by the Organization for Social Science Research in Eastern and Southern Africa (OSSREA), Addis Ababa Ethiopia. Part of the material cited here was published by OSSREA in 2005. The author wishes to acknowledge OSSREA for funding the research and giving permission to re-publish elements of the text.

## References

Ahlburg, D. A., Jensen, E. R. and Perez, A. E. (1997) 'Determinants of extramarital sex in the Philippines', *Health Transition Review*, 7(Suppl): 467–79.
Blanc, A. K. (2001) 'The effect of power in sexual relationships on sexual and reproductive health', *Studies in Family Planning*, 32/3: 189–213.
Careal, M. J., Cleland, J. G. and Ingham, R. (1994) 'Extramarital sex: implications of survey results for STD/HIV transmission: AIDS impact and prevention in developing world: demographic and social science perspectives', *Health Transition Review*, 4: 153–72.

Chinaglia, M., Tun, W., Mello, M., Insfran, M. and Diaz, J. (2008) 'Assessment of risk factors for HIV infection in female sex workers and men who have sex with men at triple boarder area of Cuidad del Este, Paraguay', *Horizons Project Final Report*, Washington DC: Population Council.

Decosas, J., Kane, F., Anarfi, J. K., Sodji, K. D. and Wagner, H. U. (1995) 'Migration and AIDS', *The Lancet*, 346: 826–28.

Fapohunda, B. M. and Rutenberg, N. (1999) *Expanding Men's Participation in Reproductive Health in Kenya*, Nairobi: African Population Policy Research Centre.

Flournoy, R. and Yen, I. (2004) *The Influence of Community Factors on Health: An Annotated Bibliography*, Policy Link and California Endowment. Online. Available from: www.policylink.org/pdfs/AnnotatedBib.pdf (accessed 15 January 2009).

Foglia G., Sateren, W. B., Renzullo, P. O., Bautista, C. T., Langat, L., Wasunna, M. K., Singer, D. E., Scott, P. T., Robb, M. L. and Birx, D. L. (2007) 'High prevalence of HIV infection among rural tea plantation residents in Kericho, Kenya', *Epidemiology and Infection*, 136: 694–702.

Gupta, G. R. and Weiss, E. (1993) 'Women's lives and sex: implications for AIDS prevention', *Culture, Medicine and Psychiatry*, 17: 399–412.

Hallman, K. (2004) *Socioeconomic Disadvantage and Unsafe Sexual Behaviour among Young Women and Men in South Africa*, Population Working Paper No. 190. New York: Population Council.

ILO (2001) *An ILO Code of Practice on HIV and AIDS*, Geneva: International Labour Organization and World Bank.

Lehrer, E. L. (2004) 'Religion as a determinant of economic and demographic behaviour in the United States', *Population and Development Review*, 30(4): 707–26.

Liyala, P. K., Biomndo, J., Davis, W., Odonde, G. D., Shanks, K. M., Wasunna, N. M. and Mason, C. (2000) 'Baseline epidemiology in a cohort of tea plantation workers and dependants in Kericho, Kenya', paper presented at XIII International Conference on AIDS, Durban, South Africa.

Lurie, M. N., Williams, B. G., Zuma, K., Mkaya-Mwamburi, D., Garnett, G., Sturm, A. W., Sweat, M. D., Gittelsohn, J. and Abdool Karim, S. S. (2003) 'The impact of migration on HIV-1 transmission in South Africa: a study of migrant and nonmigrant men and their partners', *Sexually Transmitted Diseases*, 30(2): 149–56.

Mason, K. O. (1994) 'HIV transmission and the balance of power between men and women: a global view', *Health Transition Review*, 4: 217–40.

McQuillan, K. (2004) 'When does religion influence fertility?', *Population and Development Review*, 30(1): 25–56.

Ondimu, K. N. (2005) *Risky Sexual Behaviors among Tea Plantation Workers in Kenya*, Addis Ababa, Ethiopia: Organization for Social Science Research in Eastern and Southern Africa.

Philipson, T. and Posner, R. A. (1995) 'On the macroeconomics of AIDS in Africa', *Population and Development Review*, 21: 835–48.

Pison, G., Le Guenno, B., Lagarde, E., Enel, C. and Seck, C. (1993) 'Seasonal migration: a risk factor for HIV in rural Senegal', *Journal of Acquired Immune Deficiency Syndrome*, 6(2): 196–200.

Republic of Kenya (2003) *Kericho District Development Plan 2000–2010*, Nairobi: Ministry of Planning and National Development.

Sateren, W. B., Foglia, G., Renzullo, P. O., Elson, L., Wasunna, M. K., Bautista, C. T. and Birx, D. L. (2006) 'Epidemiology of HIV-1 in agricultural plantation residents in

Kericho, Kenya: preparation for vaccine feasibility studies', *Journal of Acquired Immune Deficiency Syndromes*, 43(1): 102–6.

Sen, G. and Ostlin, P. (2007) *Unequal, Unfair, Ineffective and Inefficient Gender Inequity in Health: Why it Exists and How we Can Change it*, Geneva: Final Report to WHO Commission on Social Determinants of Health.

Smith, D. J. (2003) 'Imagining HIV/AIDS: morality and perceptions of personal risk in Nigeria', *Medical Anthropology*, 22(4): 343–72.

Tibandebage, P. and Mackintosh, M. (2005) 'The market shaping of charges, trust and abuse: health care transactions in Tanzania', *Social Science & Medicine*, 61(7): 1385–95.

UN (2005) *Population Development and HIV/AIDS with Particular Emphasis on Poverty: The Concise Report*, United Nations, Department of Economic and Social Affairs.

# Chapter 13

# Young sex workers in Ethiopia

## Linking migration, sex work and AIDS

*Lorraine van Blerk*

Since the emergence of the AIDS pandemic across sub-Saharan Africa, associations have been made between HIV transmission and the ways in which migration and sex work are connected. Much of the early literature emerging from studies conducted in East Africa in the 1980s and 1990s focused attention on sex work and HIV (Kishindo 1995; Walden *et al.* 1999; Gysels *et al.* 2001). This early literature concentrated on male mobility as a key vehicle for transmission of HIV where employment-related migration was viewed as one of the main reasons for men engaging with the services of sex workers while away from home. This encompassed the short- to medium-term migration patterns of particular workers such as truck drivers, who would use sex workers while travelling along trading routes between major ports and cities, and soldiers and sailors who regularly engaged with sex workers while stationed away from home (Omara-Otunnu 1987; Wood 1988; Larson 1990; Cohen 1999; Gysels *et al.* 2001; Varga 2001). In addition, those engaged in longer-term migration, such as male migration throughout southern Africa to the South African gold and diamond mines have also been connected with sex workers (Campbell 2000).

More recently, women's migration has been highlighted as an important factor although this was previously hidden within the literature. For example, Elder (2003) highlights how migrant women transgressed the spatial laws of South African apartheid that restricted their movement and moved into migrant worker hostel locations to provide sexual services to migrant men. Zuma *et al.* (2003) found that migrant women in South Africa were more likely than non-migrant women to engage in risky sexual behaviour, including sex work or transactional sex, had lower condom use and had higher HIV prevalence rates. Female migration for employment has also been identified in the literature as part of the feminisation of the labour force within the global economy. For example, in Lesotho the garment industry is one of the major factors influencing rural to urban female migration and is causing an increasing influx of rural migrant women into urban and peri-urban areas in search of employment. Many of these women are single or living away from home resulting in an increase in the number of sexual partners they have and a rise in HIV prevalence rates (ALAFA 2008). Although this does not conclusively suggest that poor pay and limited employment opportunities is resulting in migrant women entering into sex work to supplement their income, single migrant women have been found to be more likely to engage in sex with multiple partners and have higher HIV prevalence rates than the national average.

This suggests that women who engage in sex work are more likely to be migratory, often moving into towns from rural areas and resorting to sex work as an alternative to formal employment. However, Campbell (2000) identifies that the literature has generally portrayed sex workers as non-migratory, positioning them either as locally resident women or noting that they congregate in towns along trading routes or near to male employment. Despite this, sex workers are a mobile population which may influence HIV transmission in very direct ways (van Blerk 2007). This chapter therefore considers the links between sex work and migration through exploring the particular movements of sex workers themselves as part of the mobile transmission of HIV. The chapter begins by outlining the research process, highlighting the methods used before considering in more detail the nature of sex work in Ethiopia. The focus is on the impact of migratory pathways into sex work for rural young people and the nature of their subsequent movements on HIV transmission. The chapter concludes by calling for sex worker migration patterns to be more closely linked to HIV transmission and for policy to re-consider the ways in which sex workers are educated regarding HIV and AIDS.

## The study

The research discussed in this chapter is drawn from a project exploring the socio-spatial lives of young sex workers in Ethiopia. Enquiry took place in two cities in Ethiopia with relatively large transient populations: Addis Ababa, the capital city and Nazareth, the regional capital for Oromia district and a major entertainment centre located on the trade route between the capital and the port at Djibouti. The research was conducted in these sites to access a range of sex work occupations for teenage girls as this varies between places. For example, a larger proportion of young sex workers were found to be engaging in bar work in Nazareth, while in Addis Ababa more were found working as streetwalkers. Sixty girls, who were currently engaged in commercial sex[1] as part of their work either as bar workers (41%), streetwalkers (37%) or red-light area workers (22%), participated in this research. The girls were aged between 14 and 19 years (with a mean age of 17 years). These categories are loosely applied and include variations in the work undertaken. For example, street walkers included those girls who walk the streets and those who stood at particular places for accessing clients, while bar workers included those who work in small drinking places as well as larger bars in poor neighbourhoods, and red-light workers included those who work from brothels or small rooms with or without red lights. It is worth noting here that red-light workers are the most constrained in terms of their mobility, while bar girls and streetwalkers have freedom to move around the city to access clients and to travel further afield, which has major implications for the issues discussed in this chapter.

Young women were mainly accessed through drop-in centres although a snowballing technique was also employed to reach those who did not attend these. To overcome problems of language and cultural interpretation, I worked closely with a local translator and spent considerable time with the girls at the centres to develop rapport. I also employed a variety of qualitative methods in which the impact of my own involvement was minimised including discussions, mapping and photo diaries (see Young and Barrett 2001). This combination of methods was useful for triangulation purposes and was followed up with semi-structured interviews to elicit more detailed information about the young women's lives.

## Migration into urban areas

Despite the historical high status attached to women who provided sexual ser-vices to prominent men in Ethiopian society (most notably the women who tra-velled with the emperor's camp in the middle ages – see Pankhurst 1974), sex work now has a stigmatised reputation and is felt to bring shame on a family if a member engages in this type of work. It is viewed as antithetical to the position of women in contemporary Ethiopian society as homemakers and as subservient to their husband's authority (Pankhurst 1994). For this reason, the young sex workers in this study stressed that it is impossible for girls to begin sex work while living in the same district as their families. The work they were doing would become quickly known and their parents would no longer be able to arrange marriages for them, bringing shame to the family. Therefore all the girls that participated in the research had migrated to the districts where they now sought employment and aimed to keep their work hidden.

Genet (aged 17 years) and Zenash (aged 18 years) were two friends who shared a room in one of Addis Ababa's well-known sex worker locations. They walked the streets at night looking for work, at the same time sub-letting their room to a group of street youths. Both girls came from Addis Ababa and have not migrated far. However, they both moved from villages on the outskirts of the city to their current location because of problems at home. In each case they were accused of bringing shame on their families because they had engaged in sexual relations with boyfriends, and were thrown out of the home. They now engage in sex work or 'business' to obtain income. As Genet said, 'Once a parent finds out you have had sex [outside marriage] they tell you to leave and you are on your own ... That is how I ended up here doing business'.

Although this localised migration into other areas within or close to a city can result in young people engaging in sex work, many more are migrating to the city from rural areas (van Blerk 2009). The majority of the girls who participated in this study had moved to either Addis Ababa or Nazareth from the poverty-stricken regions of the wider rural landscape. This migration occurred for several reasons and sex work was almost always a consequence of this movement, rather than a direct reason for it. The young women spoke of coming to the city to find employment because their families could not afford to support them any longer and opportunities are limited for rural girls with low levels of formal education. They are generally restricted to informal employment such as domestic work, which can be arduous and low paid, or service sector employment in bars and coffee shops, which is unpaid and relies on tips. As Beti explained, these latter two forms of work often result in girls engaging in sex work to earn supplementary income:

> I started working as a maid but I couldn't make any money to send home and the owners were always beating me and saying bad things about me ... By doing business I can now send money to help my family
>
> (Beti, aged 16, Nazareth)

Others left home because of problems they faced in their family and home lives, or to escape cultural practices such as female circumcision. Arranged marriages are still common in many rural areas and several young women noted that they had actively sought an opportunity to leave home rather than be forced to marry someone they did not know or did not want to marry. In some cases prospective husbands were significantly older than the girls. Others had married and left because their marriage had failed or in a few cases they had been forced to marry under Telfa, a cultural practice that still remains in rural Ethiopia. In this system a man abducts a woman and once it is known that a girl has been taken it is presumed she is no longer a virgin and her family are forced into allowing her to be married to her abductor.

Sometimes the desire to move to the city resulted in girls being tricked or persuaded into moving only to find that there is no employment for them or that they have been brought to engage in sex work. A number of young women, like Ani, mentioned that they had gone to the city with a bar owner or red-light room owner who had talked about life in the city during a visit to their home village. Others mentioned they had been persuaded to leave home by a friend or relative who had returned from the city and appeared to be living a glamorous lifestyle:

> My family do not have money, they are very poor. As I am the eldest I had to get married but I did not want to marry so I left with a woman who came to our village promising work in the coffee board. When I got to Addis I realised I had to engage in business to survive and support my family.
>
> (Ani, aged 16, Addis Ababa)

The migration of rural girls to the cities in search of better opportunities and employment has important implications for HIV transmission. Alene *et al.* (2004) have reported that rural youth, although they may be sexually active, are not sufficiently engaged in prevention strategies and that condom use is low among the rural population. There are few health services to alert girls in rural areas to sexually transmitted infections and their prevention (van Blerk 2007), and generally those young women who do migrate do not move with the specific idea of starting sex work. Many are ill informed about the health implications of this type of work and some, such as Kalkidan, are inexperienced when they first begin sex work:

> I come from Derezeit. When I lived there I did not know about men or sex but my family arranged for me to marry a man I did not know so I left
>
> (Kalkidan, aged 18, Nazareth)

## AIDS and mobility

Despite the limited research on sex workers' mobility in the African context, research in other settings has demonstrated that sex workers may be highly mobile (Day and Ward 2004). In this study, mobility played a large part in the daily lives of the young women and was central to the ways in which HIV and sex work were linked. Mobility processes here include girls' movement around the cities in which they worked as well as movement between towns and cities that could involve short- or longer-term moves. Although the girls' experiences of mobility processes varied, so too did the reasons for their mobility.

### Concealing status

Sickness was identified as a key reason movement to new places to engage in sex work. Such movement was generally connected to a fear of being identified as HIV positive and therefore unable to attract clients in their current location. For example, Aster had moved to Nazareth from Addis Ababa to do business because she suspected that she might be HIV positive and changes to her health and appearance were raising suspicion. Aster attracted a lot of clients through bar work despite repeated bouts of sickness but stated that she had had to move towns to continue working because her ill health had resulted in weight loss and the other girls were beginning to suspect she was HIV positive. She changed location so that she could continue working and sending money back to her family. Similarly, Abeba moved from Nazareth to another town because ill health had made clients suspicious of her. However, although she told everyone she would return to her rural village and live with her aunt, close friends knew that instead she was going to look for business in another town where no one knew her.

Such mobility may have implications for the transmission of HIV since young women may move to conceal their suspected HIV status rather than seek testing and treatment. In part, this is due to stigma, a lack of available information and poor access to health services (van Blerk 2007) but it is also due to a lack of alternative employment. Berhane (aged 16 years), for example, explained that while she knew she was HIV positive (although she had not been tested) she felt that 'there is nothing else for me to do so I must continue in this life', whilst Tibiliz (age 18) explained 'I know I am HIV positive but I still do business. I tried to stop but there is no-one to help me'.

In some cases the need to move because of a positive HIV status was forced upon young women when clients, aware of their status, became violent towards them. Tibiliz said she had to move when the other girls found out that she was HIV positive and one of them told her regular client her status, and he became angry, threatening to beat her:

> I went to be tested and told my close friend, but the others found out and told my [regular] client so they could steal him away from me. He was angry and wants to beat me, so I must go to another place to do business.
>
> (Tibiliz, aged 18, Nazareth)

The links between mobility, HIV and AIDS can, however, be subtler as young women talked of moving to avoid the stigma of their employment. Amerat (aged 14 years) explained that 'People around us get to know our business. They treat us as though we are garbage, some even consider us as though we are animals ... so I prefer not to stay in once place too long'. As she indicated, it is the shame associated with sex work that creates stigma.

### Unknown transporters of the virus

Mobility around the city or migration to a new location can occur for a variety of reasons, none of which is directly related to HIV or AIDS, but this movement can have an impact on the diversity of clients the girls have contact with, in turn making the potential for HIV transmission greater. Difficult interactions with clients can make sex encounters especially risky for both parties. These include clients refusing to use condoms, cutting or splitting condoms because they do not want to use them[2] and violent interactions (cf. van Blerk 2009). Further, the combination of sex work and alcohol consumption, particularly for bar girls and those in red-light areas where the sale of alcohol takes place alongside sex work, can result more frequently in unprotected sex. Stating that 'You know to be drunk means to be dead [contract HIV]. We can't control ourselves and clients can have sex without condoms', Genet suggests that unprotected sex can lead to a greater risk of contracting HIV. Despite this, girls frequently reported being encouraged to drink in the bars and drinking houses where they worked.

Young women engaged in movement around the city generally because they were having difficulties in their present location. For streetwalkers, this was usually because the police were harassing them, or they had had an argument with a client or another girl and did not want to be found, or because they were having difficulty getting work in that area. For bar girls, and to a lesser extent red-light area workers, localised movement resulted mainly from a disagreement with the bar/room owner. On a few occasions, the girls reported that their movement to a new area of the city for work purposes had arisen because they had developed a relationship with a client. By moving to work in another location, the girls felt they were able to separate their work from home.

Respondents mentioned engaging in longer distance moves both because they were looking for excitement or extra work, and this enabled them to see other parts of the country. Similarly to Agustin's (2007) work, albeit in a different cultural context, sex work may be seen as a 'transportable' form of employment that can be taken to other locations. For example, at the time of the research Kalkidan (18) had recently returned to Nazareth after a four-month visit to Addis Ababa because business had been slow in her bar and she wanted some excitement. She had visited Addis Ababa once before on a similar trip and had enjoyed being in the capital city. However, Kalkidan did not want to stay there permanently and preferred to return to the bar where she worked in Nazareth. Others chose to travel according to the seasons as they felt this is the most lucrative way to see the rest of their country. As respondents explained, girls travel to different areas depending on the local harvest such as coffee or onions because the larger markets attract farmers and brokers to the area.

## Conclusions

In conclusion, this chapter has sought to highlight the direct and indirect ways in which HIV and mobility/migration may interconnect in the lives of young Ethiopian women sex workers. In understanding HIV-related vulnerability and prevention, it is wrong to assume that it is only client mobility that influences HIV transmission. Young sex workers in countries such as Ethiopia may be highly mobile and this mobility can increase vulnerability and may increase the possibility of inadvertent transmission to others. Policy and practice must reconsider the role of migration and mobility for sex workers and the impact this may have on the transmission of HIV. In addition, given that mobile populations can link together urban and rural contexts it is important for policy to consider the efficiency of education programmes in rural areas and how they might reach young girls before they migrate to urban centres as well as how education and HIV prevention initiatives can best be developed for migrant traders who travel into the seasonal markets from remote locations.

## Notes

1  Although it is acknowledged that sex work definitions can be complex, particularly in poor communities where sex may be exchanged for income or other needs at times of hardship, this paper focuses specifically on girls who exchange sex for cash with a variety of (mainly unknown) men as their main source of livelihood.
2  Some girls suspected that clients who had contracted sexually transmitted infections including HIV blamed the sex workers for their infection and split the condoms they used as a form of revenge.

# References

Agustin, L. (2007) *Sex at the Margins: Migration, Labour Markets and the Rescue Industry*, London: Zed Books.

ALAFA (2008) *HIV Sero-Prevalence Study Report*, ALAFA: Maseru.

Alene, G., Wheeler, J. and Grosskruth, H. (2004) 'Adolescent reproductive health and awareness of HIV among rural high school students, North Western Ethiopia', *AIDS Care*, 16(1): 57–68.

Campbell, C. (2000) 'Selling sex in the time of AIDS: the psycho-social context of condom use by sex workers on a Southern African mine', *Social Science & Medicine*, 50(4): 479–94.

Cohen, D. (1999) *Socio-economic Causes and Consequences of the HIV Epidemic in Southern Africa: A Case Study of Namibia*, Issue Paper No. 31, UNDP HIV and Development Programme.

Day, S. and Ward, H. (2004) *Sex Work, Mobility and Health in Europe*, London: Routledge.

Elder, G. (2003) *Hostels, Sexuality, and the Apartheid Legacy: Malevolent Geographies*, Athens and Ohio: Ohio University Press.

Gysels, M., Pool, R. and Bwanika, K. (2001) 'Truck drivers, middlemen and commercial sex workers: AIDS and the mediation of sex in south west Uganda', *AIDS Care*, 13(3): 373–85.

Kishindo, D. (1995) 'Sexual behaviour in the face of risk: the case of bar girls in Malawi's major cities', *Health Transition Review*, 5(Suppl): 153–60.

Larson, A. (1990) 'The social epidemiology of Africa's AIDS epidemic', *African Affairs*, 89: 5–25.

Omara-Otunnu, A. (1987) *Politics and the Military in Uganda*, London: Macmillan.

Pankhurst, H. (1994) *Gender, Development and Identity: An Ethiopian Study*, London: Zed Books.

Pankhurst, R. (1974) 'The history of prostitution in Ethiopia', *Journal of Ethiopian Studies*, 12(2): 159–78.

van Blerk, L. (2007) 'AIDS, mobility and commercial sex in Ethiopia: implications for policy', *AIDS Care*, 19(1): 79–86.

——(2008) 'Poverty, migration and sex work: youth transitions in Ethiopia', *Area*, 40(2): 245–53.

——(2009) 'Negotiating boundaries: bar girls and sex work in Ethiopia', *Unpublished manuscript, contact author for details*.

Varga, C. (2001) 'Coping with HIV/AIDS in Durban's commercial sex industry', *AIDS Care*, 13(3): 351–65.

Walden, V., Mwangulube, K. and Makhumula-Nkhoma, P. (1999) 'Measuring the impact of a behaviour change intervention for commercial sex workers and their potential clients in Malawi', *Health Education Research*, 14(4): 545–54.

Wood, W. (1988) 'AIDS North and South: diffusion patters of a global epidemic and a research agenda for Geographers', *The Professional Geographer*, 40: 266–69.

Young, L. and Barrett, H. (2001) 'Adapting visual methods: action research with Kampala street children', *Area*, 33(2): 141–52.

Zuma, K., Gouws, E., Williams, B. and Lurie, M. (2003) 'Risk factors for HIV infection among women in Carletonville, South Africa: migration, demography and sexually transmitted diseases', *International Journal of STD & AIDS*, 14: 814–17.

# Chapter 14

# Labour migration and HIV risk in Papua New Guinea

*Holly Wardlow*

Not much more than a decade ago, many in the small community of scholars, activists, and health practitioners working on HIV in Papua New Guinea hoped that the epidemic might remain confined to Port Moresby, the national capital – at least long enough for an effective prevention strategy to be mounted. Road infrastructure is undeveloped in the country and it is impossible to travel far from Port Moresby except by plane or boat. Few roads lead out of the city, and none of them link to another urban centre or to the Highlands Highway, the main artery bisecting the country from east to west. With the capital city so divorced from the rest of the country, and with 85 per cent of the population living in rural areas, it was hoped that the epidemic could be stemmed before it had a chance to become generalized.

At the same time, it was also known that Papua New Guinea shares many characteristics with countries that have a high prevalence of HIV, including an economy dependent on mining; contraction of economic opportunity, particularly in rural areas; a very young population; severe deterioration of basic health services, including closure of rural aid posts and health centres in the 1990s (Duke 1999); and high rates of gonorrhoea, syphilis, and other sexually transmitted infections, with some studies showing long delays in treatment seeking (Passey 1998; Hughes 2002). In addition, although mobility in and out of Port Moresby is constrained, the main arteries in the rest of the country connect seven of the provincial capitals to each other, and many unpaved roads link rural communities to these main arteries. Moreover, since at least the 1960s, plantation labour recruitment policies, population relocation schemes, and the development of the mining industry have helped create a highly mobile male population.

The supposition that HIV might stay confined to urban centres did not adequately take into account this longstanding high level of mobility. Similarly, social science research in Papua New Guinea has overlooked the issue, and has not yet systematically focused on the relationship between labour migration and HIV risk. There are, however, older anthropological, geographical, and historical literatures on labour-related mobility in Papua New Guinea. This chapter attempts to show the relevance of this literature for understanding current HIV risk, and for generating important research questions. For example, the chapter discusses the way in which quite different regional histories of population movement were created during the Australian colonial era when some communities in Papua New Guinea were given strong incentives – such as free seedlings and infrastructure improvements – to become cash croppers, while others were deliberately cultivated as labour-exporting regions. These different histories of mobility, in turn, gave rise to different patterns of sexual networking, and thus of HIV vulnerability (Thornton 2008). Different regional histories of migration also generated different cultures of migration – that is, community-specific ways of investing meaning in the act: whether migration is frowned upon or a source of prestige; what a family will expect when a migrant returns home; and how this varies by age, gender, and marital status. For example, in some communities with a long and intensive history of male out-migration, working away from home has become a typical stage in the male life-course and a formative part of masculinity.

The chapter begins with an overview of HIV in Papua New Guinea, then discusses the specific economic development policies, both colonial and more recent, that have shaped labour migration in the country. Three points emerge: (1) one consequence of uneven development has been that some communities have been targeted as sources of labour for other regions, and thus that a stint of labour migration has become a normative stage in masculine development in these communities; (2) population relocation schemes that were meant to alleviate land pressures were short-sighted in planning for migrants' descendants, thus leading to economic insecurity, particularly for women; (3) mining company labour policies, particularly their privileging of local communities as sources of labour, contribute to particular patterns of sexual networking and HIV-related risk.

## Papua New Guinea and HIV/AIDS

With a population of almost six million, Papua New Guinea occupies the eastern half of the island of New Guinea and some surrounding smaller islands. It gained independence from Australia in 1975, and although one of its official national languages is English, it is home to more than 850 indigenous languages. Much of the terrain consists of steep mountains and dense tropical rain forest, making infrastructure development and social service delivery difficult.

The first case of HIV in Papua New Guinea was diagnosed in 1987, but prevalence appeared to remain low until the mid 1990s, with reported new cases increasing only from 17 to 69 between 1989 and 1994. The Papua New Guinea National AIDS Council was established in 1997, and since that time HIV testing and case reporting have expanded and improved, resulting in a dramatic increase in reported cases. How much of the annual increases are due to actual increases in new infections and how much are due to the expansion of testing is debated. As the 2008 United Nations General Assembly Special Session (UNGASS) report states:

Until quite recently, very limited HIV surveillance data gave a poor understanding about the progress of the epidemic and its geographic distribution across the country ... Since the Port Moresby General Hospital was the only site providing testing for HIV in the country for almost 10 years, over 50 per cent of all reported HIV infections come from the National Capital District ...

(UNGASS 2008: 22)

The recent establishment of more than 60 Voluntary Counselling and Testing centres around the country has revealed HIV-positive cases in all provinces, and although surveillance still needs improvement (some health centres fail to submit reports, or do so with basic information missing, such as gender and age), the Papua New Guinea National AIDS Council estimates a 2009 HIV prevalence of 2.56 per cent (98,757 cases), with a projected increase to more than 5 per cent prevalence by 2012 (UNGASS 2008). Eighty-five per cent of cases are located in rural areas, a dramatic departure from what had been assumed to be a largely urban-based epidemic. Heterosexual sex is the primary mode of transmission, with cases distributed equally between men and women, although with women infected at younger ages than men. The most thoroughly documented aspect of HIV vulnerability is acute gender inequality that includes women's economic dependence on men, their isolation from family and other social support once married, and pervasive sexual violence (National Sex and Reproduction Research Team and Jenkins 1994; Wardlow 2006, 2009; Hammar 2008; Lepani 2008).

## The Highlands Labour Scheme

By the 1930s, the demand for labour on Australian colonial plantations in Papua New Guinea had outstripped the supply available from coastal communities (Ward 1990). Thus, when the New Guinea mountainous interior – which had been thought to be uninhabited – was found to be densely populated, plantation owners were eager to tap into this new source. For a variety of reasons, including the advent of World War II, a formal system for recruiting highlands men to work on coastal plantations was not, however, put in place until the 1950s. Plantation owners and colonial administrators disagreed about labour recruitment strategies, with the former advocating minimal restrictions so that they could quickly obtain the bodies needed to rehabilitate their estates, and the latter 'anxious to ensure that exploitation of workers did not take place and to avoid deleterious effects of recruiting upon the home areas' (Ward 1990: 279).

Because the highlands populations had only recently been 'discovered', they were seen by the colonial administration as both immunologically and culturally vulnerable. The administration was well aware of the pattern of de-population that had occurred due to newly introduced infectious diseases in many areas of the Pacific (Jolly 1998; Denoon et al. 2000). Thus, when it was finally implemented in 1950, the Highland Labour Scheme was relatively protectionist in nature: employers were not allowed to recruit in the highlands; only government officers on patrol in rural areas were permitted to inform people about the possibility of working on coastal plantations, and the rations, wages, and expected medical care were all outlined in detail (Ward 1990).

The scheme was successful for almost two decades, and by 1974, when the programme ended, more than 100,000 men had been recruited through it to work on lowland plantations. However, the initial areas of recruitment, Goroka and Mount Hagen, were also the areas where highland smallholders were establishing their own coffee fields (Stewart 1992). Growing coffee at home was much preferred to plantation work elsewhere; thus, in order to find workers for lowland plantations, the colonial administration extended its labour recruitment to new areas, with the consequence that some regions, Southern Highlands Province in particular, were cultivated as labour pools for plantations located in other provinces (Harris 1972; Connell 1997). This pattern continued even after the scheme came to an end; migration data from 1982, for example, show that in some Huli communities in Southern Highlands Province, approximately 45 per cent of the men between the ages of 20 and 39 had out-migrated (Lehmann 2002).

One result of this long involvement in labour migration is that it has become an expected part of masculine experience among the Huli. Research I conducted with Huli married men in 2004 showed that many associated labour migration with the possibility of sexual adventure, and many asserted that they became sexually experienced while working at plantations or mines. They also described how migrant male friendships are forged and maintained through drinking, buying sex from female sex workers, joking about sexual liaisons, and sharing information about sexual partners (Wardlow 2007, 2008, 2009). In some cases, these activities are less an expression of *esprit de corps* and more a kind of peer pressure that reinforces hierarchical relationships between employed men. As one man said:

> It was his idea—he was my boss and I was the driver. He said, 'Let's go around and find some women. I'll pay for some food and I'll pay for the guest house.' So I did this the first time because I was with him ... Lots of working men do this—they pressure each other to go drink and have sex with prostitutes. It was especially hard for me because I worked as the driver, so they expected me to drive them to hotels and other places and it was hard for me to say no.

In this region, the history of labour migration has thus become integral to masculine experience, and has facilitated a construction of masculinity that includes both sexual sociality – in the sense that men often go out as a group to drink alcohol and find sexual partners – and sexual autonomy, in the sense that working men demonstrate their independence from traditional community norms through extramarital liaisons. Moreover, this construction of masculinity is not necessarily situational and does not necessarily end once the migrant comes home: men learn and cultivate a particular style of masculinity through their migrant experiences, and sometimes bring it back home with them, continuing to search out sex workers while in the company of male peers. One dimension of migration and HIV risk that merits more attention is thus how labour migration and masculinity, including masculine sexuality, can be mutually constitutive phenomena.

## Palm oil relocation schemes

Based on research in East Sepik Province, a mainland province with a somewhat different set of factors shaping migration, Curry and Koczberski (1998, 1999) similarly argue that migration has become a 'rite of passage' for Wosera men. Some regions within this province also have a relatively long history of out-migration due to colonial era population redistribution policies: in this case, in the 1960s the Australian administration was concerned that the Wosera were suffering from high population density and poor land. They were thus targeted for relocation to the north coast of West New Britain, an island province with sparse population and fertile soil. The colonial government acquired land from local communities, subdivided it into blocks, and rented the blocks to the relocated migrants with 99 year leases. The blocks were typically leased for the specific purpose of cultivating cash crops, initially coconut and cocoa, with oil palm rapidly overtaking these. In order to attract both corporate and small-holder investment, the 'nucleus estate system' was established whereby small-holders (also called outgrowers) supply oil palm fruit to mills operated by a central plantation. There are now at least five large nucleus estate-outgrower oil palm projects in Papua New Guinea, and oil palm has overtaken coffee as the most valuable cash crop.

Koczberski and Curry suggest that the descendants of the initial migrants now find themselves in a socially and economically precarious situation. First, there were far more migrants than anticipated: migrants now make up almost 30 per cent of the West New Britain population (Koczberski and Curry 2004). This is largely because of chain migration, in which families and friends follow those who have already migrated. Visitors sometimes stay with their relocated kin for as long as two years: the lease-holding families find it difficult to ask them to leave, in part because they hope that generosity to visitors will enable them re-establish claims to land if they return 'home'. Although the initial lease-holding migrants may have moved as a family, their visitors tend to be men engaged in two- or three-year contracts:

> The young man on his first trip away typically stays first with relatives on a block or squatter settlement. Subsequently, he may move onto a plantation and be housed in the single men's quarters. If he tires of work, the blocks

and squatter settlements offer respite from plantation work ... Thus, a visitor living for several years in West New Britain may make several moves during his stay, resulting in a continual flow, mainly of men, between the blocks, squatter settlements and plantation estates.

(Curry and Koczberski 1998: 35)

Curry and Koczberski's research does not address men's sexual networking in this context or whether extramarital sexuality has become a normal part of the Wosera male migration experience, as seems to be the case for Huli men. However, other research suggests that some oil palm plantations have become sites for transactional and commoditized sexual liaisons. For example, the *mama lus frut* scheme (loose fruit mothers; certainly not the best choice of name), in which women gather and sell the oil palm fruit that is left on the ground after the main harvest, has become associated with sex work. Some observers report that male harvesters will deliberately leave more fruit on the ground for women to collect in exchange for sex.[1]

Another factor that likely contributes to HIV risk at oil palm sites is that resettlement schemes failed to make provisions for the children of the initial lease holders. The initial single-family blocks of land have become multiple-household blocks supporting the original owner, his married sons, and their families. The oil palm income – as well as the land set aside for growing food – is now shared by all, an unsustainable situation that has created family conflict and food insecurity. This situation is exacerbated by two factors. First, most migrant families cannot go 'home' again. They most often come from land-short areas, and Curry and Koczberski (1999) demonstrate that the migrants' generous hosting of visitors is not, in fact, enough to maintain their rights to land in their sending communities. Second, the West New Britain communities hosting the migrants now feel that they were inadequately compensated by the government when their land was appropriated for oil palm resettlement schemes. This resentment is often expressed through harassment – and even forced eviction – of migrants, despite the fact that the migrant lease holders are there legally (Koczberski and Curry 2004). In short, in some cases, land resettlement schemes have resulted in second-generation settlers who have no rights to land at 'home' and quite tenuous rights to land in the provinces in which they were born. Social science research suggests that this pattern of first generation migration, followed by second generation economic insecurity, landlessness, and ethnic conflict, creates 'HIV risk ecologies' (Lyons 2004; Beer 2008).

## Mineral development and mine site labour policies

The third point to emerge from a review of the labour migration literature concerns the well-known HIV risk associated with mines and their environs. Most of the qualitative or ethnographic models that explain this risk are based on examples from South Africa, and focus primarily on mine workers' HIV vulnerability (Moodie 1994; Campbell 1997, 2003). However, it would be a mistake to assume that mining town risk ecologies are the same the world over. Different national mineral development policies may result in different patterns of composition of mining workforces, as well as in differences in the way the workforce is housed, and in how labour time is organized. All these factors can, in turn, have an impact on the sexual networking patterns of both miners and others in the community. This is not to say that mining towns in Papua New Guinea are somehow radically different from those in South Africa: certainly many factors – women migrating to mine sites to sell sex, for example – are similar. Nevertheless, an analysis of the Porgera Joint Venture (PJV) gold mine in Papua New Guinea suggests that the policy particulars of the national context do matter. For example, in 2006, based on voluntary testing, HIV prevalence among PJV employees was approximately the same as the national average of approximately 2 per cent, while prevalence for the Porgera community as a whole, also based on voluntary testing, was much higher at 8 to 10 per cent (*Corporate Social Responsibility News*, 30 November 2007).[2] If these figures are accurate, it would seem there is an important difference between miners' vulnerability and that of the rest of the community. Furthermore, community HIV prevalence in Porgera, a remote mountain town, is higher than that in most cities.

While numerous factors surely shape the HIV risk ecology at Porgera, Papua New Guinea's mineral development policy, and its consequences for PJV's workforce, may explain part of the difference. Papua New Guinea differs from most mining-dependent countries in one important respect: the Land Act of 1962 states that all land not appropriated prior to the Act is legally held by traditional landowning groups. The consequence is that 97 per cent of land is under customary communal ownership. This distinguishing characteristic is important because it requires a mining company to identify – and sign a compensation and royalties agreement with – the relevant local landowners in order to obtain a mining lease from the national government (by law the state owns subsoil resources, and thus all mining leases must be negotiated with the state). Thus, as Benedict Imbun notes, 'local people enjoy an unprecedented upper hand in negotiating for their interests with mining companies—and have more influence than the government' (Imbun 2000: 101). Furthermore, the terms of the PJV mining lease were negotiated when another mine, the Panguna copper mine on Bougainville island, was being violently shut down by local landowners who were angry about environmental damage and inadequate compensation. As a result, 'landowners at Porgera ... gained a better share of royalty payments, greater compensation payments, promises of significantly improved infrastructure and more participation in decision-making' (Connell 1997: 140; see also Filer and Imbun 2004; Golub 2007).

Construction of both open pit and underground mining operations at Porgera began in 1989, and in 1992 the mine produced 1,485,077 ounces of gold, making it the third most productive gold mine in the world at that time (Golub

2006). One demand made by Porgera landowners was that they be given pre-ference in hiring. The resulting PJV employment policy is relevant for under-standing HIV risk because it also specifies that local employees may not receive mining camp accommodation: only expatriates and non-Porgeran national employees may live in the mine's residential compounds, and then only when they are on duty. Local employees, who make up approximately one-third of the mine's workforce of more than 2000 persons, commute daily from villages near the mine. (Or at least this is what they are thought to do. It is possible that some employees stay with town-based kin rather than making the daily commute back to the village, a potentially important factor for understanding sexual networking in Porgera.) Moreover, PJV's employment policy is that non-local employees maintain a roughly two-week-on/two-week-off schedule in which they work from six am to six pm when they are on duty. Thus, in theory, even non-local employees are separated from their families for only two weeks at a time. Again, there are no data about where these employees actually go during their time off. My preliminary research indicates that at least some of them go to Mount. Hagen and other urban areas rather than returning home during their time off. This is also likely to have implications for sexual networking patterns.

Thus, in contrast to the model of mining and HIV risk in South Africa, it is not the case in Papua New Guinea that most workers come from afar and are separated from their wives and communities for months or years at a time. The long separation of miners from their families, and the failure of mining compa-nies to provide family housing, have long been emphasized as fundamental fac-tors contributing to HIV and other sexually transmitted infection risk at South African mines. Randall Packard, for example, comments that in 1913, when William Gorgas was invited to inspect conditions on the Rand and make recommendations regarding tuberculosis and syphilis prevention, he advised that mineworkers be housed with their families instead of in all-male barracks (Pack-ard 1989:78). The advice was not taken. Ninety years later Catherine Campbell wrote:

> Migrant workers travel to the mines from a range of areas in and around South Africa, where they are housed in single-sex hostels, which sometimes house as many as 12 or 18 men in a room ... Within this all-male context, a thriving commercial sex industry has sprung up. Impoverished women find accommodation in informal shack settlements on mine perimeters from where they sell sex and alcohol to the miners who form the major con-sumers in a complex informal economy.
>
> (Campbell 2003:12–13)

The problem of long-term separation from family is central to this model of HIV vulnerability: as Daan Brummer comments, 'High-risk behaviour such as sex with multiple partners is not solely the result of migration. It is also the result of alienation, of loneliness, of being separated from family and regular partners' (Brummer 2002:9). It would appear, however, that the Porgeran HIV risk ecology may be structured somewhat differently because many of the employees are local landowners who are expected to live at home. Why other Porgera area residents are at disproportionate HIV risk is another piece of the puzzle that urgently demands further research.

## Conclusion

People are often surprised to hear that HIV and AIDS are serious problems in Papua New Guinea. AIDS seems like such a modern problem, and Papua New Guinea is still seen by many people as one of the few remaining places in the world where small, isolated societies continue to carry out their traditional customs. However, while Papua New Guinea's colonial history may have been relatively brief and benign, it ushered in rapid and dramatic changes, including the mobilization of people, especially men, for labour on plantations and in mines. And while researchers have not yet focused on the role of labour migration in the production of HIV risk environments in Papua New Guinea, there is much to be learned from the existing migration literature. This literature suggests that labour migration has become an expected stage in masculine development in labour-exporting communities. Further, this stage is associated with sexual adventure and with membership in male peer groups whose solidarity is maintained in part through finding female sexual partners together. At the same time, it is important to examine the particulars of each case. It is possible, for example, that the composition and organization of the labour force at Papua New Guinea mine sites – in which many labourers are local and other labourers can live at home two weeks every month – reduce sexual networking and thus HIV risk, at least for the labourers themselves, if not for others in mining communities. Labour migration is certainly not the only factor creating HIV risk environments in Papua New Guinea, nor should it be studied in isolation. The ways in which migration, ethnic conflict, and gendered violence intersect and amplify HIV risk at sites of economic development is also an important question. Nevertheless, our current understanding of sexual networking in these economic enclaves is inadequate. If nothing else, then, this chapter has identified urgent areas for new research.

## Notes

1 See www.wrm.org.uy/bulletin/123/Papua.html (accessed September 17, 2008).
2 Some of this discrepancy may be due to the efforts that Barrick, the current owner of the Porgera Mine, has put into HIV and AIDS awareness, condom availability, confidentiality for HIV-positive employees, and informing employees of their rights to antiretroviral treatment and to continued employment. Barrick does not have before and after epidemiological data, and so it is difficult to know the impact of these policies on HIV prevalence among employees of the mine.

# References

Beer, B. (2008) 'Buying Betel and Selling Sex: Contested Boundaries, Risk Milieus, and Discourses about HIV/AIDS in the Markham Valley, Papua New Guinea', in L. Butt and R. Eves (eds) *Making Sense of AIDS: Culture, Sexuality, and Power in Melanesia*, Honolulu: University of Hawai'i Press.

Brummer, D. (2002) *Labour Migration and HIV/AIDS in Southern Africa*, Pretoria: International Organization for Migration.

Campbell, C. (1997) 'Migrancy, Masculine Identities and AIDS: The Psychosocial Context of HIV Transmission on the South Africa Gold Mines', *Social Science & Medicine*, 45(2): 273–81.

——(2003) *Letting Them Die: Why HIV/AIDS Prevention Programmes Fail*, The International African Institute in association with Oxford, Indiana University Press and Double Storey.

Connell, J. (1997) *Papua New Guinea: the Struggle for Development*, New York: Routledge.

Curry, G. and Koczberski, G. (1998) 'Migration and Circulation as a Way of Life for the Wosera Abelam of Papua New Guinea', *Asia Pacific Viewpoint*, 39(1): 29–52.

——(1999) 'The Risks and Uncertainties of Migration: an Exploration of Recent Trends amongst the Wosera Abelam of Papua New Guinea', *Oceania*, 70: 130–45.

Denoon, D., Mein Smith, P. and Wyndham, M. (2000) *A History of Australia, New Zealand, and the Pacific: The Formation of Identities*, Oxford and Malden, Massachusetts: Blackwell Publishing.

Duke, T. (1999) 'Decline in Child Health in Rural Papua New Guinea', *Lancet*, 354: 1291–94.

Filer, C. and Imbun, B. (2004) 'A Short History of Mineral Development Policies in Papua New Guinea', Resource Management in Asia-Pacific Working Paper No. 55, Research School of Pacific and Asian Studies, Canberra: Australian National University Press.

Golub, A. (2006) 'Who is the "Original Affluent Society"? Ipili "Predatory Expansion" and the Porgera Gold Mine, Papua New Guinea', *The Contemporary Pacific*, 18(2): 265–92.

——(2007) 'From Agency to Agents: Forging Landowner Identities in Porgera', in J. Weiner and K. Glaskin (eds) *Customary Land Tenure and Registration in Australia and Papua New Guinea: Anthropological Perspectives*, Canberra: ANU E-Press.

Harris, G.T. (1972) 'Labour Supply and Economic Development in the Southern Highlands', *Oceania*, 43: 123–39.

Hammar, L. (2008) 'Fear and Loathing in Papua New Guinea: Sexual Health in a Nation under Siege', in L. Butt and R. Eves (eds) *Making Sense of AIDS: Culture, Sexuality, and Power in Melanesia*, Honolulu: University of Hawai'i Press.

Hughes, J. (2002) 'Sexually Transmitted Infections: a Medical Anthropological Study from the Tari Research Unit 1990–91', *Papua New Guinea Medical Journal*, 45(1–2): 128–33.

Imbun, B. (2000) *Industrial and Employment Relations in the Mining Industry*, Port Moresby: University of Papua New Guinea Press.

Jolly, M. (1998) 'Other Mothers: Maternal Insouciance and the Depopulation Debate in Vanuatu and Fiji', in K. Ram and M. Jolly (eds) *Maternities and Modernities: Colonial and Postcolonial Experiences in Asia and the Pacific*, Cambridge: Cambridge University Press.

Koczberski, G. and Curry, G. (2004) 'Divided Communities and Contested Landscapes: Mobility, Development and Shifting Identities in Migrant Destination Sites in Papua New Guinea', *Asia Pacific Viewpoint*, 45(3): 357–71.

Lehmann, D. (2002) 'Demography and Causes of Death among the Huli in the Tari Basin', *Papua New Guinea Medical Journal*, 45: 51–62.

Lepani, K. (2008) 'Mobility, Violence, and the Gendering of HIV in Papua New Guinea', *The Australian Journal of Anthropology*, 19(2): 150–64.

Lyons, M. (2004) 'Mobile Populations and HIV/AIDS in East Africa', in E. Kalipeni, S. Craddock, J. Oppong and J. Ghosh (eds) *HIV and AIDS in Africa: Beyond Epidemiology*, Malden, Massachusetts: Blackwell Publishing.

Moodie, T. D. (1994) *Going for Gold: Men, Mines and Migration*, Berkeley, California: University of California Press.

National Sex and Reproduction Research Team and Carol Jenkins (1994) *National Study of Sexual and Reproductive Knowledge and Behavior in Papua New Guinea*, Papua New Guinea Institute of Medical Research Monograph #10, Goroka: Institute of Medical Research.

Packard, R. (1989) *White Plague, Black Labour: Tuberculosis and the Political Economy of Health and Disease in South Africa*, Berkeley, California: University of California Press.

Passey, M. (1998) 'Community Based Study of Sexually Transmitted Diseases in Rural Women in the Highlands of Papua New Guinea: Prevalence and Risk Factors', *Sexually Transmitted Diseases*, 74: 120–27.

Stewart, R. (1992) *Coffee: the Political Economy of an Export Industry in Papua New Guinea*, Boulder, Colorado: Westview Press.

Thornton, R. (2008) *Unimagined Community: Sex, Networks, and AIDS in Uganda and South Africa*, Berkeley, California: University of California Press.

UNGASS (2008) *United Nations General Assembly Special Session on HIV and AIDS Country Progress Report*, Papua New Guinea National AIDS Council Secretariat and Partners.

Ward, R. G. (1990) 'Contract Labour Recruitment from the Highlands of Papua New Guinea, 1950–74', *International Migration Review*, 24(2): 273–96.

Wardlow, H. (2006) *Wayward Women: Sexuality and Agency in a New Guinea Society*, Berkeley, California: University of California Press.

——(2007) 'Men's Extramarital Sexuality in Rural Papua New Guinea', *American Journal of Public Health*, 97(6): 1006–14.

——(2008) '"She Liked It Best when She was on Top": Intimacies and Estrangements in Huli Men's Marital and Extramarital Relationships', in W. Jankowiak (ed.) *Intimacies: Love and Sex across Cultures*, New York: Columbia University Press.

——(2009) '"Whip Him in the Head with a Stick!": Marriage, Male Infidelity, and Female Confrontation among the Huli', in J. S. Hirsch, D. J. Smith, H. Wardlow, S. Parikh, H. M. Phinney and C. A. Nathanson *The Secret: Love, Marriage and Infidelity*, Nashville, Tennessee: Vanderbilt University Press.

# Chapter 15

# Migration, men's extramarital sex and the risk of HIV infection in Nigeria

*Daniel Jordan Smith*

In southeastern Nigeria, mobility and migration are key strategies for economic livelihood. As the basis for subsistence shifts from agriculture to wage labour and participation in commerce, and as people's aspirations grow to include consumption of modern commodities, urban-influenced lifestyles and relatively expensive education for their children, few households can manage their financial needs without work-related migration. For the Igbo ethnic group that dominates the region, as for many African people, migration strategies commonly involve maintaining a household in a rural place of origin while some members of the family embark on economically motivated migration of varying durations – from a few days to many years (Geschiere and Gugler 1998; Chukwuezi 2001; Gugler 2002). When migration divides families into rural and urban households, most typically, but certainly not uniformly, it is a husband/father who migrates and a wife/mother who stays in the village to raise the children and supervise rural economic activities such as farming and small-scale trade.

The necessity and pace of economic migration grew in Nigeria during the same period as the emergence of the country's HIV epidemic. While Nigeria has avoided the catastrophically high infection rates characteristic of southern Africa and parts of east Africa, with an adult seroprevalence of about four per cent and Nigeria's population of over 140 million people, more than two and a half million citizens are estimated to be infected, the third highest absolute number of any country in the world (UNAIDS 2008). In many world regions where the most common form of transmission is heterosexual, increasing attention has been focused on the risk of marital transmission (UNFPA, UNAIDS and UNIFEM 2004; Hirsch *et al.* 2007). In particular, the reality of gender inequality and of widespread double standards with regard to men's and women's sexuality have led many researchers to explore the social contexts and pathways by which married men might infect their wives through their involvement in unprotected extramarital sex (Hirsch *et al.* 2007; Parikh 2007; Wardlow 2007; Phinney 2008).[1] The urgency of this research and the implications of these findings are amplified by the emphasis in global HIV prevention on the 'ABC approach' (Abstain, Be Faithful, Use Condoms), which touts the protective benefits of fidelity for people involved in sexual relationships, a promise upon which married women with cheating husbands cannot rely. In Nigeria, moralistic messages that extol abstinence and fidelity as avenues to HIV prevention are common, but so is male infidelity (Smith 2003, 2007, 2008; Mitsunaga *et al.* 2005).

Married women's vulnerability to HIV infection from unfaithful spouses appears to be exacerbated by the changing nature of marriage itself. In south-eastern Nigeria, as in many parts of the world, younger couples increasingly value choosing their own life partner, often based on a notion of romantic love (Smith 2001; Hirsch 2003; Hirsch and Wardlow 2006). While one might expect that modern marriages are beneficial to women because they choose their part-ners themselves and because the personal relationship between husband and wife is central to the quality of a marriage, my research challenges this view. In fact, as the conjugal relationship becomes more privileged as a locus of emotional investment vis-à-vis other social ties, Igbo women lose some forms of leverage with their husbands. In the context of men's continued pursuit of extramarital sexual relationships, women's power vis-à-vis their husbands is a crucial factor in navigating the risk of HIV infection. High rates of mobility and migration both increase men's opportunities for extramarital sex and complicate women's abilities to protect themselves.

In this chapter, I focus on the specific contexts of Igbo men's mobility and migration that enable and even encourage extramarital sexual behaviour. The description and analysis of the influence of mobility and migration on men's behaviour is situated in relationship to other social factors that shape men's desires to cheat on their wives. My findings emphasize the ways in which men's infide-lity must be understood not simply as a natural biological desire or as individual ethical failing, but also as the product of structural opportunities and social circumstances. After explaining men's behaviour, I will briefly examine how migration that splits spouses for extended periods of time intersects with changes in marriage itself to affect married women's responses to their husbands' infidelity.

## Study background

The material in this chapter is the result of a recent study undertaken in two communities in Igbo-speaking southeastern Nigeria, where I have worked and conducted research since 1989.[2] Project regions included the semi-rural com-munity of Ubakala in Abia State and the city of Owerri in Imo State. Ubakala is made up of 11 villages and has a total resident population of approximately 24,000 people. Most households rely economically on a combination of farming, trading, employment and remittances from migrants. The community is about six miles from the town of Umuahia, and everyday life is increasingly affected by the close orbit with an urban centre. Furthermore, the vast majority of adults in Ubakala have lived at least a year or more in one of Nigeria's many cities, and at any given time more than half the people who consider Ubakala their 'home' are living outside the community, mostly in Nigeria's far-flung cities and towns.

Despite significant changes over the past several decades that have placed strains on traditional systems of social organization, ties of kinship and community remain powerful among both Ubakala residents and their migrant kin.

Owerri is the capital of Imo State and has a population of approximately 350,000 people. Many of the city's residents work as civil servants for the state government, but there are also large commercial and service sectors. The bulk of the population is made up of rural–urban migrants, most of whom retain close ties to their places of origin. As in Ubakala and across the entire southeastern region, Christianity is nearly ubiquitous in Owerri. In addition, Owerri is the home of four colleges and universities and has a student population of close to 100,000. Partly because of the concentration of tertiary institutions, the city has a reputation throughout southern Nigeria as a hub for extramarital sexual relationships.

This research draws primarily on material collected from June to December 2004, when I stayed in a household in Ubakala that included a married woman, several children, and a mostly absent migrant husband, and in Owerri with a newlywed couple who were rural–urban migrants. Marital case studies were conducted with 20 couples, 14 residing in rural Ubakala and six residing in urban Owerri. The couples were selected opportunistically with the objective of sampling marriages of different generations and duration, couples with a range of socioeconomic and educational profiles, and, of course, people in both rural and urban settings. Interviews were conducted in three parts, generally in three sessions, each approximately 1–1.5 hours in duration. Husbands and wives were interviewed separately. Given the sensitive nature of the topics discussed, I interviewed the men and female research assistants interviewed the women. In general, men seemed to be more at ease talking about extramarital sex than women. This is probably attributable to the prevailing gender double standard, but it may have also been the case that men were more comfortable talking to me as an outsider and women were more wary of discussing such issues with the local compatriots. The first interview concentrated primarily on premarital experiences, courtship, and the early stages of marriage. The second interview examined in greater depth the overall experience of marriage, including issues such as marital communication, decision-making, childrearing, resolution of disputes, relations with family, patterns of residence and migration histories, and changes in the marital relationship over time. The final interview focused on marital sexuality, extramarital sexual relationships, and understandings and experiences regarding HIV and AIDS.

## Men's motives for extramarital sex

The prevalence of married men's participation in extramarital sex in Nigeria is well documented (Karanja 1987; Lawoyin and Larsen 2002; Mitsunaga *et al.* 2005; Smith 2007). As in many societies, people in southeastern Nigeria commonly attribute men's frequent participation in extramarital sexual relationships to some sort of innate male predisposition, and this perspective is well represented in the literature (Orubuloye *et al.* 1997). Explaining male extramarital sexual behaviour in these terms is insufficient, however, because sexual desires do not emerge or operate in a social and cultural vacuum, and because the opportunity to indulge desire is itself contingent on numerous other factors. Rather, from interviews with men about their extramarital relationships, from listening to men's conversations among themselves pertaining to these relationships and from observations of men interacting with their extramarital partners in various public or semi-public settings, a number of patterns in the motives for and the social organization of men's extramarital sex became apparent.

Three factors emerged as particularly important for explaining male infidelity: (1) socioeconomic status, (2) involvement in predominately male peer groups that encourage or reward extramarital sexual relations, and (3) mobility and migration – the main focus of this chapter. Before concentrating on mobility and migration as structural factors that facilitate male infidelity, a brief explanation of the intertwining influences of socioeconomic status and male peer groups on married men's motivations for extramarital sex is necessary. Both factors are interconnected with the effects of mobility and migration.

Men frequently view extramarital relationships as arenas for the expression of economic and masculine status. Indeed, it is necessary to understand the intertwining of masculinity and wealth, and gender and economics more generally, to make sense of the most common forms of infidelity in southeastern Nigeria. In popular discourse, the most common form of economically driven extramarital relationships is said to be so-called 'sugar daddy' relationships. A closer look at these relationships suggests that they are much more complicated than portrayed in the stereotypical image of rich men exchanging money for sex with impoverished girls (Smith 2002; Cornwall 2002; see Hunter 2002 and Luke 2005 for similar perspectives focused in other sub-Saharan African settings). Typical female participants in these sugar daddy relationships are not the truly poor, but rather young women who are in urban secondary schools or universities, and who seek and represent a kind of modern femininity. They are frequently educated, almost always highly fashionable, and while their motivations for having a sugar daddy may be largely economic, they are usually looking for more than money to feed themselves. For married men, the pretty, urban, educated young women who are the most desirable girlfriends provide not only sex, but the opportunity, or at least the fantasy, of having more exciting, stylish, modern, and 'high-class' sex than what they have with their wives.

Based on my sample, men with money appear to have easier access to and more frequent extramarital sex. But poorer men engage in extramarital sex as well, and their relationships with female partners also typically include some form of transaction, whether it is paying a sex worker or giving gifts to a girlfriend, albeit at a lower financial level than more elite men. While infidelity knows no class boundaries, it is nevertheless true that in contemporary southeastern Nigeria many married men who have younger girlfriends are asserting a brand of masculinity wherein sexual prowess, economic capability, and modern sensibility are intertwined.

Masculinity is created and expressed both in men's relationships to women and in their relationships with other men (Connell 1995; Smith 2008). In male-dominated social settings such as social clubs, sports clubs, sections of the marketplace, and particular bars and eateries, Igbo men commonly talk about their girlfriends, and sometimes show them off. These male-dominated contexts build on a much longer history of sex-segregated social organization in Igbo society, where kinship groups and village associations meet in gender-separate forums, church activities and seating are distinctly divided between men's and women's sections, and forms of labour are highly sex-segregated (Uchendu 1965). In predominantly male contexts, men encourage and reward extramarital relationships.

Further, the ways in which men discuss, share, encourage and regulate each other's extramarital behaviour are part of how men create and navigate intimacy with each other. Seeing men encourage and reward each other for extramarital sex is an everyday experience in masculine spaces. Men will compliment each other on the beauty of their lovers and listen admiringly to stories about recent sexual exploits. While sexual virility is one aspect of masculinity that is performed and reinforced when married men show off younger unmarried lovers, demonstrating socioeconomic status is equally central to men's public self-presentations. Although my friends commonly complained among themselves about the consumptive demands of their girlfriends – symbolized most recently by the growing expectations for mobile phones – it was also true that the capacity to provide these things was precisely part of what men were demonstrating to themselves and their peers in keeping expensive girlfriends (Smith 2006).

## Mobility, migration and men's extramarital sex

While the rewards of extramarital sex provided by male peers reinforced the motives for many men's infidelity, mobility and migration emerged as the most common structural variables that created specific opportunities for extramarital liaisons. Further, in the contexts of men's mobility and migration, the social significance of proving masculine economic capability and the sway of male peer pressure appear to be amplified. Mobility and migration not only take men away from their wives and from the watchful eyes of their home communities, they also bring them into the orbit of social forces that encourage infidelity.

Of the 20 men interviewed for the marital case studies in urban Owerri and rural Ubakala, 14 reported having extramarital sex at some point during their marriages, and of the six who said they had not engaged in extramarital sex, four had been married less than five years. Approximately half of all the cases of extramarital relationships described in the interviews occurred in situations where work-related migration was a factor. Two common patterns could be discerned, one related to longer-term migration and the other to men's mobility in contexts where they reside with their wives. In contemporary Nigeria it is increasingly common that men take their wives and children with them when work sends them to live in faraway places for long periods of time. But as indicated above, many households maintain a dual residence strategy, where wives and children stay in the village to ease the costs of children's education, enable continued farming of family land and maintain important ties in a place of origin. As a result, many men live apart from their wives for months and years at a time, with trips home only weekly or monthly, and sometimes less frequently, depending on the distance and available economic means.

Several men told stories of extramarital relationships undertaken in this context, and they frequently attributed their behaviour to the opportunities and hardships produced by these absences. For example, Obi, a 43-year-old merchant who has a business selling cosmetic products in Lagos and visits his wife and children in rural Ubakala 8–10 times per year, described his extramarital relationships as a consequence of migration: 'I live most of the time apart from my wife. Without her presence there are chances and I have needs'. As with many men whose work-related migration takes them far from their wives for extended periods of time, Obi described a longer-term extramarital relationship in which his lover performed many of the tasks typically provided by a wife, such as cooking and washing clothes. In exchange, women like Obi's lover often have the status of what has frequently been described in the literature as an 'outside wife' (Karanja 1987). But like most men who admitted cheating on their wives, Obi was careful to point out that the relationship never threatened, in his mind, his commitment to his marriage and family. 'My family still comes first', he said. In response to a question about whether he would ever consider divorcing his wife for his lover, Obi responded: 'Absolutely not. She [his long-term Lagos-based lover] helps me manage the difficulty of my situation, but in our culture marriage is permanent. There is no question of divorce'.

While many men who spent extended periods of time separated from their wives as a consequence of work-related migration described relatively stable and enduring extramarital partnerships, men also frequently spoke of contexts of male peer-group sociality that encouraged more fleeting sexual relationships. Men living without their families in the city commonly spend some of their non-work hours in the company of other migrant men, often in bars, restaurants and hotels that cater to this population. In these settings younger single women are commonly present (in some settings this includes sex workers) and available to men who are willing to spend some of their cash cultivating a relationship. It is in these settings that the connections between men's desire to assert their economic capability and their concerns with their social reputations among male peers intersect with the loneliness, freedom and opportunities created by migration to make extramarital sex appealing, easy and common.

Although work-related migration is an important factor in creating opportunities for male infidelity, it is nevertheless true that men who live with their wives also engage in extramarital sexual relationships. But even in these circumstances, men's mobility proved to be a major feature in understanding the dynamics of male infidelity. Many aspects of modern life – especially co-educational schooling and women's increasing participation in the urban labour force – have created trends toward greater integration of men's and women's social worlds. Nevertheless, as emphasized above, sex-segregated social life remains common. Men and women spend most of their work and leisure time with people of the same gender. Part of this sex-gender system is a double standard that allows married men considerably more mobility than married women. In interviews, both men and women routinely indicated that a woman needs to seek permission from her husband to undertake anything other than the routine mobility of going to the farm, the market or church, while a man is free to engage in a much wider range of movement, including socializing and drinking with other men and going to town. A man only feels obliged, at best, to 'inform' his wife of his movements, but certainly does not feel compelled to ask permission. It is in this context of relative male mobility – particularly in male-dominated social settings that include alcohol and a population of unmarried women – that men who reside with their wives sometimes commence extramarital sexual relationships.

## The meaning of infidelity and consequences for condom use

Before turning to the question of how married Igbo women respond to their husbands' cheating, it is necessary to comment on two other features of men's infidelity: men's perceptions of the significance of their relationships and their likelihood of condom use. The first strongly affects women's reactions to their husbands' cheating and the second has serious implications for the risk of HIV infection. Perhaps the most significant finding from the interviews with men, but also from much more widely overheard conversations that men had about extramarital sex, was the fact that almost no men articulate infidelity as being an indication of a lack of commitment to their marriages and families. While most men recognized that their wives might become jealous or angry and might feel hurt if they discovered that their husbands cheated, almost uniformly, men indicated their firm commitment to their marriages. In men's minds, this loyalty took the form of maintaining responsibility for provisioning the household, always according their wives due respect in their public role as wife, and never allowing their extramarital relationships to result in divorce. To the vast majority of men, a deep commitment to marriage and the practice of infidelity were by no means incompatible realities.

With regard to condom use, men's reports of their practices in extramarital relations were variable, but also quite consistent with what is reported in the literature not only for sub-Saharan Africa, but much more widely. While some men reported regular condom use and others expressed disdain for the method, by far the most common pattern was that men said they used condoms for more fleeting relationships or at the beginning of extramarital affairs, but that once relationships became more stable, condom use diminished. In addition, because many men sought to distance their extramarital sexual behaviour from the more stigmatized practice of paying for commercial sex, it seemed apparent that condom use was inhibited by its association with risky sex and immoral partners, a finding that I also observed among the unmarried population in southeastern Nigeria, and which has been found in many other cultural contexts where condoms are promoted to prevent HIV infection (Smith 2003).

## Married women's responses to men's infidelity

For married women who discover or suspect that their husbands are cheating, the fact that men do not see – and indeed society in general does not see – men's infidelity as a fundamental threat to marriage complicates women's responses. It is certainly true that most Igbo women experience male infidelity as a violation. Further, in the context of the rise of so-called modern marriage, where women have a greater say in the choice of their spouses and where the ideal of romantic love is increasingly valued as a basis for marrying, younger women feel particularly aggrieved by the emotional betrayal of their husbands' cheating. But the social reproductive project of marriage is still more highly valued by society – and, arguably, by most women themselves – than the ideals of love and fidelity. In this context, divorce is both stigmatizing and difficult and women risk spoiling their identities, losing regular access to their children and facing an uncertain future if they allow their discontents about men's infidelity to evolve into irreconcilable ruptures.

As a result, many women remain silent, at least publicly, about their husbands' extramarital sexual behaviour. Indeed, not a single woman in my sample acknowledged that her husband was currently cheating, even though the interviews with their husbands revealed that several women clearly knew or suspected that their husbands were unfaithful. Women's tolerance and public silence reflects both the consequences of continued gender double standards and women's calculations that in these circumstances it is more in their interest to preserve a marriage than to create major conflicts over men's infidelity. It is a thorny question as to whether women's relative tolerance makes them complicit in perpetuating men's infidelity, or whether they simply have no choice. It is certainly true that women strongly value the status of wife and mother and that in the southeastern Nigerian context men are careful to carry on their extramarital relations in a manner that preserves and tacitly respects both the institution of marriage and the public status of wifehood, insofar as this is possible. But as the ideals for marriage are changing, men's extramarital relationships and the gender double standards upon which they are founded have become increasingly problematic for many women.

The fact that women feel compelled – and to some extent are highly motivated – to stay married, even to cheating husbands, makes the possibility of protecting themselves from potential HIV infection extremely difficult. For women who suspect their husbands of infidelity, suggesting condom use for marital sex poses multiple problems. Asking for a condom may imply she does not want to become pregnant, which itself can create tension because reproduction is extremely highly valued. Perhaps worse, her request may be interpreted as indicating that she suspects not only that her husband is cheating, but that the type of extramarital sex he is having is risky, which in the Nigerian context connotes that he may have had sex with a prostitute. What is more, the meaning of her request may be inverted by her spouse and turned against her with an accusation that it is she who is being unfaithful. Responding to a question about whether his wife had ever asked him to use a condom, a 34-year-old father of three exclaimed:

> How can she? Is she crazy? A woman asking her husband to use a condom is putting herself in the position of a whore. What does she need a condom with her man for, unless she is flirting around outside the married house?

All of these possibilities have become more highly charged in the era of AIDS, when sexual immorality is associated with a deadly disease.

The ultimate irony is that for women in the most modern marriages, where the conjugal relationship is primary and romantic love is often an explicit foundation of the relationship, the possibility of confronting a man's infidelity or insisting on condom use is even more difficult. In such marriages, a woman challenging her husband's extramarital behaviour or asking for a condom may be undermining the very basis for the marriage and threatening whatever leverage she has with her husband by implying that the relationship itself has been broken. The secrets and silences that result can exacerbate married women's risk of HIV infection.

## Conclusion

Most government and donor-supported approaches to preventing HIV infection in Nigeria, like elsewhere, emphasize educating individuals to adopt behaviours – notably, abstinence, fidelity and condom use – that are meant to be protective. Yet mounting evidence demonstrates that knowledge about HIV and about preventive actions often does not translate into effective behaviour change. In the face of data that suggests marital transmission is an important mode of infection in countries with large heterosexually driven epidemics, policy-makers, programme personnel and scholars have all begun to recognize that abstinence and fidelity are not effective protective strategies for people in marriages where partners are unfaithful. Women appear to be particularly powerless to protect themselves, both because male infidelity seems to be more common and because multiple aspects of marital dynamics and gender inequality make it nearly impossible for women to request, much less insist on, condom use with their husbands.

While married women's vulnerability is increasingly acknowledged, little research has focused on the social contexts that produce men's infidelity. Commonly, men's extramarital sexual behaviour is attributed to biological factors such as evolutionary predispositions, hormones, or generic notions about sex drive. More socially attuned perspectives typically acknowledge and often lament the double standards that are the product of systematic gender inequality. But few accounts examine married men's sexual behaviour from a more structural perspective, situating infidelity in broader political-economic and social-relational contexts. In this chapter, I have presented evidence to argue that male infidelity in southeastern Nigeria is facilitated and powerfully shaped by livelihood strategies that require migration and by gendered social norms that encourage male mobility. The impact of migration and mobility on men's propensity to cheat on their wives is augmented by the ways that mobility and the consequent separation of husbands and wives – not only geographically but also socially – intersects with the influence of male peer groups and with the intertwining social class and masculine identity. In contexts of mobility and migration, Igbo men appear to feel even greater pressure to engage in extramarital relationships in which they simultaneously perform both masculine and economic status.

Married women's capacity to respond is inhibited not only by long-standing patterns of gender inequality, but also by newer marital ideals and practices that privilege notions of romantic love, expectations for intimacy and the relative importance of the conjugal relationship vis-à-vis other social ties. Ironically – and, from the perspective of married women's risk of HIV infection, tragically – as Igbo women have been able to exercise more choice over who they marry and as they have been able to select husbands based partly on whether they feel a romantic or emotional connection, confronting men's infidelity seems to have become even more difficult.

## Notes

1 Other researchers have justifiably questioned whether all the focus on men's infidelity and the risk of marital transmission for women obscures the extent and epidemiological consequences of married women's extramarital sexual behaviour. In particular, Lurie *et al.* (2003) have shown in a study of migration and serodiscordant couples in South Africa that a significant proportion of married women are contracting HIV infection through extramarital sex. The focus in this chapter on married men's behaviour is not meant to deny the reality that women also cheat on their husbands, though in the southeastern Nigerian context male infidelity is more common. Nevertheless, the evidence from studies that reveal women's extramarital behaviour in the context of migration only strengthens the argument here that structural factors such as migration are central to understanding the contexts of HIV risk.

2 Most of the data presented in this chapter were collected while working on a five-country comparative ethnographic study entitled 'Love, Marriage and HIV: A Multisite Study of Gender and HIV Risk', funded by the National Institutes of Health (Grant 1R01 HD 041724).

# References

Chukwuezi, B. (2001) 'Through thick and thin: Igbo rural–urban circularity, identity and investment', *Journal of Contemporary African Studies*, 19(1): 55–66.

Connell, R. (1995) *Masculinities*, Cambridge: Polity Press.

Cornwall, A. (2002) 'Spending power: love, money, and the reconfiguration of gender relations in Ada-Odo, southwestern Nigeria', *American Ethnologist*, 29(4): 963–80.

Geschiere, P. and Gugler, J. (1998) 'The urban–rural connection: changing issues of belonging and identification', *Africa*, 68(3): 309–19.

Gugler, J. (2002) 'The son of a hawk does not remain abroad: the urban–rural connection in Africa', *African Studies Review*, 45(1): 21–41.

Hirsch, J. S. (2003) *A Courtship after Marriage: Sexuality and Love in Mexican Transnational Families*, Berkeley: University of California Press.

Hirsch, J. S., Meneses, S., Thompson, B., Negroni, M., Pelcastre, B. and del Rio, C. (2007) 'The inevitability of infidelity: sexual reputation, social geographies, and marital HIV risk in rural Mexico', *American Journal of Public Health*, 97(6): 986–96.

Hirsch, J. S. and Wardlow, H. (eds) (2006) *Modern Loves: The Anthropology of Romantic Courtship and Companionate Marriage*, Ann Arbor: University of Michigan Press.

Hunter, M. (2002) 'The materiality of everyday sex: thinking beyond "prostitution"', *African Studies*, 61(1): 99–120.

Karanja, W. (1987) '"Outside wives" and "inside wives" in Nigeria: a study of changing perceptions', in D. Parkin and D. Nyamwaya (eds) *Transformations in African Marriage*, Manchester: International African Institute.

Lawoyin, T.O. and Larsen, U. (2002) 'Male sexual behavior during wife's pregnancy and postpartum abstinence period in Oyo State, Nigeria', *Journal of Biosocial Science*, 34(1): 51–63.

Luke, N. (2005) 'Confronting the "sugar daddy" stereotype: age and economic asymmetries and risky sexual behavior in urban Kenya', *International Family Planning Perspectives*, 31(1): 6–14.

Lurie, M., Williams, B., Zuma, K., Mkaya-Mwamburi, D., Garnett, G., Sweat, M., Gittelsohn, J. and Karim, S. (2003) 'Who infects whom? HIV-1 concordance and discordance among migrant and non-migrant couples in South Africa', *AIDS*, 17(5): 2245–52.

Mitsunaga, T., Powell, A., Heard, N. and Larsen, U. (2005) 'Extramarital sex among Nigerian men: polygyny and other risk factors', *Journal of Acquired Immune Deficiency Syndrome*, 39(4): 478–88.

Orubuloye, I. O., Caldwell, J. and Caldwell, P. (1997) 'Perceived male sexual needs and male sexual behavior in southwest Nigeria', *Social Science & Medicine*, 44(8): 1195–207.

Parikh, S. (2007) 'The political economy of marriage and HIV: the ABC approach, "safe" infidelity, and managing moral risk in Uganda', *American Journal of Public Health*, 97(7): 1198–208.

Phinney, H. (2008) '"Rice is essential but tiresome; you should get some noodles": *Doi Moi* and the political economy of men's extramarital sexual relations and marital HIV risk in Hanoi, Vietnam', *American Journal of Public Health*, 98(4): 650–60.

Smith, D. J. (2001) 'Romance, parenthood and gender in a modern African society', *Ethnology*, 40(2): 129–51.

——(2002) '"Man no be wood": gender and extramarital sex in contemporary southeastern Nigeria', *The Ahfad Journal*, 19(2): 4–23.

——(2003) 'Imagining HIV/AIDS: morality and perceptions of personal risk in Nigeria', *Medical Anthropology*, 22(4): 343–72.

——(2006) 'Cell phones, social inequality, and contemporary culture in southeastern Nigeria', *Canadian Journal of African Studies*, 40(3): 496–523.

——(2007) 'Modern marriage, men's extramarital sex, and HIV risk in Nigeria', *American Journal of Public Health*, 97(6): 997–1005.

——(2008) 'Intimacy, infidelity, and masculinity in southeastern Nigeria', in W. Jankowiak (ed.) *Intimacies: Love and Sex across Cultures*, New York: Columbia University Press.

Uchendu, V. (1965) *The Igbo of Southeast Nigeria*, Fort Worth: Holt, Reinhart and Winston.

UNAIDS (2008) *Epidemiological Fact Sheet on HIV and AIDS, Nigeria 208 Update*, Geneva: UNAIDS.

UNFPA, UNAIDS and UNIFEM (2004) *Women and HIV/AIDS: Confronting the Crisis*, New York: UNFPA, UNAIDS & UNIFEM.

Wardlow, H. (2007) 'Men's extramarital sexuality in rural Papua New Guinea', *American Journal of Public Health*, 97(6): 1006–14.

# Chapter 16

# Migration, detachment and HIV risk among rural–urban migrants in China

*Xiushi Yang*

By the end of 2007, China was home to an estimated 700,000 people living with HIV or AIDS (State Council AIDS Working Committee Office and United Nations Theme Group on AIDS 2008). While statistics appear to indicate a slowdown in new infections, sexual transmission has replaced drug-related transmission to become the dominant route of HIV infection (56.9 per cent of new infections in 2007) and a decisive factor in the future course of the epidemic in China (Merli *et al.* 2006). In 2007 alone, more than 356,000 cases of gonorrhoea and syphilis were officially reported nationwide, indicating widespread unsafe sex among China's 1.3 billion population. This, and the spread of commercial sex in China (van den Hoek *et al.* 2001; Parish *et al.* 2003; Pan *et al.* 2004) will likely continue to fuel the epidemic growth of sexually transmitted infections (STIs) and HIV unless effective measures are taken to reduce unsafe sexual behaviours.

While the causes of the spread of unsafe sex and HIV transmission are likely to be complex and multifaceted, increasing rural–urban migration may be one of the main catalysts. Although sources vary, the temporary migrant population, which constitutes the majority of rural–urban migrants in contemporary China, was estimated to have grown from 11 million in 1982 to 79 million in 2000 (Liang and Ma 2004), and most recent national estimates put the number at almost 132 million (NBS 2008). The uprooting of so many men and women may create conditions that are conducive to sexual risk behaviour and the spread of sexually transmitted infections. Indeed, the rapid and continuing spread of HIV in China is arguably best understood in the context of social and economic changes associated with increasing migration in the country (Smith and Yang 2005).

Recent research in China has provided empirical evidence for the role increasing migration plays in the spread of unsafe sex (Anderson *et al.* 2003; Hu *et al.* 2006; Yang 2006), but has also suggested significant differences between male and female migrants (Yang and Xia 2008). While most studies have focused on informal, temporary (*non-hukou*) migration in post-reform China, no research has actually compared it to formal, permanent (*hukou*) migration. Thus, little is known as to whether rural–urban migration in general or particular types of migration are conducive to unsafe sex and consequently STIs including HIV.

Using the recent migration and HIV literature in China to compare the two types of rural–urban migration, I argue here that the social/residential detachment associated with non-permanent migration is the key mechanism that renders non-permanent migrants more vulnerable to sexual risk behaviour than both long-term migrants and non-migrants.

## Background

In the early 1950s, a series of laws and regulations were implemented to formerly establish a nationwide system of household registration (*hukou*) in China to regulate rural–urban migration (Cheng and Selden 1994; Wang 2004). Under this system, everyone was born with an agricultural or non-agricultural *hukou*, determined by his/her parents' *hukou* status. A non-agricultural *hukou* entitled its holders to urban residence and the government provision of social services and benefits, including non-agricultural employment, free medical services, and pension. An agricultural *hukou*, by contrast, was associated with rural residence; its holders were supposed to be self-sufficient and entitled to few government-provided services and benefits. While there were considerable advantages to holding a non-agricultural *hukou*, permanent changes in residence/type of *hukou* were strictly controlled. Only under special circumstances, such as government-approved non-agricultural job transfers, attending colleges, and job assignment of college graduates, would a permanent change be granted. By attaching employment and social services to possession of a local *hukou* while limiting the circumstances under which a change of *hukou* could be granted, local governments exercised tight control over migration.

While one could in theory, just move, changes of residence not officially approved meant that migrants could not obtain a local *hukou* in the place of destination; people without a local *hukou* were not able to find a job, buy food and other necessities, or have access to social services. With no market alternatives in pre-reform China, it was almost impossible for migrants to survive economically and socially in urban places if their relocations were not officially approved.

In addition to residence regulation and its associated resource allocation, *hukou* in China plays an important role in maintaining social order and behavioural conformity to societal norms and rules. As the administrator of the *hukou* system, every police station has a full-time officer responsible for getting to know registered residents under its jurisdiction, including whereabouts and current main activities. These watchful eyes in turn help to maintain social order and exercise the formal and normative social controls over individual behaviour (Wang 2004).

For almost three decades up until the 1980s, the *hukou* system functioned as planned. Despite huge differences in standards of living between rural and urban areas, migration, especially rural–urban migration, was effectively controlled. Residential stability in turn led to stable communities where residents knew each other and strangers were easily identified and closely monitored. Therefore, it was considered the most important factor explaining the low crime rate and relative absence of drugs and extra-marital sex in pre-reform China (Whyte and Parish 1984; Troyer *et al.* 1989).

However, profound structural changes since the early 1980s have greatly undermined the effectiveness of the *hukou* system in regulating migration. In urban areas, more relaxed employment policies and legalization of private businesses have resulted in an increasingly differentiated employment structure, which places more and more labour force outside the control of government. The result is a dualistic division of jobs between state or large collective enterprises and small collective units or private forms of labour activities (Fan 2002). With few exceptions, jobs in the latter are often rejected by urban youth because they offer no job security, few benefits, and little social prestige. This situation has forced firms to turn to the rural–urban migrants for their labour needs. Concurrently, reforms in rural areas have dismantled the collective control of agricultural production. Land is allocated and cultivated by individual households, and non-agricultural activities are promoted. More efficient household-based production has resulted in hundreds of millions in rural surplus labour (Roberts 1997).

These changes mean that although permanent residency and rural to urban *hukou* change remains strictly controlled and highly selective, both the legal and market barriers to living in cities without a local permanent *hukou* have been considerably reduced (Yang 1993; Liang and Ma 2004; Wang 2004; Yang and Xia 2008). Not surprisingly, an increasing number of rural residents have responded to the new opportunities by migrating to cities even though they still cannot satisfy government-stipulated conditions for a permanent change in residence. This new and growing form of rural–urban migration is commonly referred to as temporary migration (*renkou liudong*) in China, precisely because it involves no change in migrants' permanent residence. Such rural–urban non-*hukou* migration has grown rapidly, becoming a key strategy among rural households in reallocating their labour (Roberts 1997).

Whether increasing migration is the cause or not, the crime rate has been on the rise and drugs and prostitution have resurfaced in China since the 1980s. In particular, social norms concerning love, marriage, and sexual relationships in general have undergone considerable change (Zhang *et al.* 1999; Farrer 2002; Yan 2003). The divorce rate is on the rise and non-marital sex is increasingly tolerated and practised, particularly among younger generations. Although technically illegal, sex work is widespread and readily available in cities throughout the country. Within this context of changes in attitudes towards sexual relationships, the uprooting and transitory lifestyle of so many young migrant men and women has led to serious concerns about the potential for the spread of risky sexual behaviours and HIV (Hu *et al.* 2006; Yang 2006; Li *et al.* 2007; Yang *et al.* 2007). Rural–urban non-*hukou* migrants are widely considered a key risk population and a tipping point in China's fight against the expansion of the HIV epidemic (Anderson *et al.* 2003).

## Migration and sexual risk of HIV

Two general theoretical perspectives help to establish the link between rural–urban migration and unsafe sex. The first is the social control perspective. Social control theory (Gibbs 1982; Black 1984) posits that every society develops formal and normative structures through which it regulates individual behaviour toward conformity to societal norms and rules (Coser 1982). Having unsafe sex with multiple partners can be pleasurable; individuals may have the natural tendency toward the behaviour, but refrain from it because they fear the negative sanctions that may result from violating societal norms and rules.

A second general theory that helps link migration to sexual behaviour is the social isolation perspective (Wilson 1987). Social isolation is characterized by a lack of sustained interaction with mainstream individuals and institutions. When disconnected from the mainstream society, individuals are deprived of exposure to positive role models for social behaviour. They are also more likely to feel lonely and depressed, which makes them vulnerable to substance abuse and/or sexual risk behaviours as a coping mechanism.

In both perspectives, rural–urban non-*hukou* migrants may be more vulnerable than the *hukou* migrants. First, the lack of a local permanent *hukou* in cities may pose a barrier to temporary migrants' full integration into the urban communities where they live and work. Despite market alternatives, state/government jobs, subsidized housing and medical services, and pensions all remain highly desired, but accessible only to those with local *hukou*. Migrants without local *hukou*, have to depend on the market for their employment needs, housing, education, and all other social services, and consequently remain 'outsiders' in the urban community regardless of how long they may have been living and working there. The rural–urban divide is being transformed into a divide between the local *hukou* haves and have-nots in cities throughout China (Wang 2004).

Many rural–urban non-*hukou* migrants in China are concentrated in the margins of the urban economy and are socially, culturally, and residentially isolated from 'mainstream' society in the city. They do the dirty, dangerous, and dead-end jobs (Knight *et al.* 1999; Solinger 1999; Wang *et al.* 2002) and live with fellow villagers at the work place or in migrant communities in areas of the city characterized by overcrowding and social disintegration (Ma and Xiang 1998; Zhang 2001). Despite limited economic gains, rural–urban non-*hukou* migrants in general experience little social or cultural assimilation in the city, feel helpless, insecure, discontented, and resentful, and are prone to substance abuse and unsafe sexual behaviours (Anderson *et al.* 2003).

Most rural–urban non-*hukou* migrants leave behind families, again weakening normative controls over behaviour. Being away from spouses or regular sexual partners, non-*hukou* migrants are more likely to experience sexual frustration, which may contribute to their extra-marital or commercial sex as a way to escape loneliness, bury anxieties about family, and release sexual frustration. Thus, by detaching rural–urban non-*hukou* migrants from origin and destination communities and likely families as well, non-*hukou* migration can weaken both formal and normative social controls, norms and morality and sexual fidelity and help migrants to maintain anonymity.

## The study

Data used in the analysis come from a population-based sample survey conducted in 2003 in China's Yunnan province. The survey was part of a study funded by the US National Institute on Drug Abuse and focused on the link between migration and the HIV risk of drug use and sexual behaviours. Sample selection followed a three-stage procedure. First, confidential registries of known HIV and AIDS cases and drug users from the provincial public health and public security bureaus and estimates of non-*hukou* migrants from the 1995 mini-census were used to rank all counties/cities in the province. From the ranked list, eight counties/cities were selected, giving priority to places with a higher concentration of known HIV, drug use, and migrant population, and geographically representing the province. These criteria were then applied to rural townships and urban neighbourhoods in each of the eight selected locations and, within these, five townships and/or neighbourhoods were selected from each. This resulted in a total of 40 townships and neighbourhoods as the primary sampling units (PSUs).

In each PSU, all individuals aged 18 to 55 were listed in one of four categories: HIV positive, drug users, temporary migrants, and non-migrants (including *hukou* migrants). They were crosschecked for multiple listings. If an individual appeared in more than one category, the individual was reassigned to only one category according to the following priority order: HIV, drug user, non-*hukou* migrant, and non-migrant. For example, a non-*hukou* migrant who was also a drug user and HIV positive, was retained in the list of HIV positives and removed from the lists of migrants and drug users. Therefore, all individuals would appear in only one of the four mutually exclusive lists.

In selecting individuals, disproportionate probability sampling (Bilsborrow *et al.* 1997) was used to make sure the resulting sample would contain sufficient numbers of 'rare' populations, for example, HIV positive and drug users, but was not overwhelmed by non-migrants. A target random sample of 150 individuals from each PSU was planned and distributed as follows: 20 HIV positive, 30 drug users, 40 non-*hukou* migrants, and 60 non-migrants. In each category, sample selection started by randomly picking a person from the list and continued selecting at fixed intervals determined by the ratio between the total on the list and the target number for the category. If a list contained fewer than the target number, everyone listed was selected. Because not every PSU had the target number of subjects in all categories, the actual sample size per category varied across PSUs.

To protect the confidentiality of study participants, all sample selections were conducted by field supervisors who had undergone training in research ethics.

All study participants were combined in lists by study ID only. Interviewers and all other fieldworkers were blind to the status (category) of study participants. A master list by participant ID, sampling category, and PSU was only accessible to the project director, was used to assign a category code to all completed questionnaires and was destroyed after completion of fieldwork and data entry.

During the fieldwork, interviewers visited sampled individuals, explained to them the purpose of the study, their right to refuse, and compensation for completing the survey. If a respondent could not be reached or refused to participate, a replacement was selected randomly from the original sampling list. The overall participant refusal was low (3.4%), which was not unusual in China. The only exception was for people living with HIV, of whom almost 29 per cent were absent or refused participation. Of the original sample of 5,570, a total of 5,382 individuals consented to participate and completed a face-to-face interview. Excluding rural–rural, urban–urban, and urban–rural migrants, the remaining sample of 3,943 is used in the analysis here.

It is important to note that not all HIV-positive persons on the confidential registries used in sampling were aware of their HIV status, nor were these registries complete in recording all those who were HIV positive, drug users, and/or non-*hukou* migrants. However, the survey questionnaire contained multiple questions on HIV, drug use, and migrant status. Some hidden HIV-positive individuals, drug users, and migrants who would have been included in the non-migrant category would have revealed their respective status on the questionnaire. Still, the sample was unlikely completely representative of the entire HIV-positive, drug-using, and non-*hukou* migrant populations. The sample of persons with HIV may have been further biased due to their higher absentee/ refusal rate.

## Methods and measures

STATA software (version 9) was used to examine if and to what extent rural–urban non-*hukou* migrants differed from comparable rural–urban *hukou* migrants and non-migrants in HIV risk sexual behaviours. Because of the use of PSU and disproportionate probabilities in sampling, all analyses are further corrected for survey design and adjusted for sampling probabilities using STATA's 'svy' analysis, designed specifically for the analysis of complex survey data.

The dependent variables were two dichotomous variables and one composite index, all measuring respondents' sexual risk of HIV. The two dichotomous variables indicate whether the respondent had (1) casual sex and (2) unprotected sex with a casual partner(s) in the 30 days prior to the interview. The composite sexual risk index combined eight dichotomous (1 yes and 0 no) variables, indicating whether the respondent had casual sex, unprotected casual sex, commercial sex, multiple casual sexual partners, multiple casual sexual acts, any episodes of drinking and drug taking while having sex, and any known injection drug use sexual partner in the 30 days prior to the survey. The eight (0/1) answers are summed to form the index. Such a composite index is arguably subject to less response bias than any single dichotomous measure (Williams *et al.* 2001). It also measures the overall sexual risk of HIV. The higher the index, the higher the sexual risk of HIV of the respondent. Cronbach's alpha for the composite index with the survey data was 0.80.

The key individual variable is a four-category migrant status variable, indicating rural non-migrant, urban non-migrant, rural–urban *hukou* migrant, and rural–urban non-*hukou* migrant, respectively. All cities and officially designated towns were considered urban and townships rural. A rural–urban non-*hukou* migrant was someone who did not possess the local permanent *hukou* in the urban PSU of interview and whose permanent *hukou* was in a rural township. Respondents who had local permanent *hukou* and were born in the rural or urban PSU of the interview were defined as rural or urban non-migrants.

A number of demographic characteristics and measures of social isolation and social control were included in the multiple regression analysis to control for differences across migrant status which may have confounded the relationship between rural–urban migration and sexual risk of HIV. This also helped to ascertain if and to what extent rural–urban non-*hukou* migrants' elevated sexual risk of HIV was due to their unique demographic characteristics (i.e., selectivity) and the extent of social isolation and weakened social control.

As variables, gender, age, and marital status are self-explanatory. Education was measured using a seven-category ordinal variable, ranging from one for illiterate to seven for four years or more of college education. Social isolation was measured by a modified version of the UCLA Loneliness Scale (Russell 1996), the Center for Epidemiologic Studies Depression Scale (Radloff 1977), and an economic marginalization index. For the loneliness scale, respondents reported on a four-point scale how lonely they felt in relation to each of 20 statements, while the depression scale was based on ratings of 20 statements about the frequency of depressive symptoms experienced in the week prior to the interview. Answers to the 20 statements of the two scales were summed to form a 'loneliness' and a 'depression' scale, respectively. The economic marginalization index was constructed by first dichotomizing answers to 15 questions on employment, industry, occupation, income, and perceived working conditions and related benefits, and then summing the (0/1) answers. Cronbach's alphas were 0.80, 0.84, and 0.86 for the loneliness, depression, and economic marginalization scale/index, respectively.

Finally, weakened social control was measured by a modified version of the Attitudes toward Authority Scale (Emler 1999) and respondents' living arrangements. Respondents reported yes (1) or no (0) to their personal experience of nine events indicating disrespect for laws or use of 'deviant' ways to achieve personal ends. Answers were then summed to create the weakened social control scale. The higher the score, the more likely the respondent had behaved with disrespect for laws or deviant ways, indicating weakened social control.

Cronbach's alphas for the scale was 0.71. Living arrangements were measured by a dichotomous variable, which took the value of 1 if respondents were living alone at the time of interview and 0 if they were living with family or others. Living alone is expected to be associated with weakened social control.

## Findings

Table 16.1 presents the sample characteristics by migrant status. *Hukou* migrants appeared to comprise largely women (mostly moving to their husband's area of registration) and the better educated, while non-*hukou* migrants were on average younger, less likely to be married, and more likely to have elementary or junior high school education.

Except for economic marginalization, for which rural non-migrants scored the highest on the index, there were few differences between non-migrant groups and *hukou* migrants in the other two measures of social isolation. Non-*hukou* migrants, however, faired the worst in measures of loneliness and feelings of depression; and scored considerably higher on the economic marginalization index than *hukou* migrants.

*Table 16.1* Sample characteristics among non-migrants and rural–urban migrants

| Individual characteristics | Rural non-migrants | Urban non-migrants | Hukou migrants | Non-hukou migrants |
|---|---|---|---|---|
| *Demographic characteristics* | | | | |
| Age (mean) | 32.4 | 32.9 | 34 | 29.2 |
| Male (%) | 55 | 52 | 37.2 | 46.4 |
| Married (%) | 84.8 | 83.2 | 87.9 | 56.2 |
| Education (%) | | | | |
| Illiterate | 21.4 | 9.5 | 12.3 | 12.4 |
| Elementary | 33.4 | 25.2 | 21 | 40.7 |
| Junior high school | 35.8 | 41.1 | 28.7 | 41.2 |
| Senior high school or more | 9.4 | 24.2 | 38.1 | 5.7 |
| *Social isolation* | | | | |
| Economic marginalization (mean) | 11.2 | 9.7 | 8.4 | 10.9 |
| Loneliness (mean) | 37.8 | 36.6 | 37.8 | 40.9 |
| Depression | 33.4 | 32.9 | 33.6 | 35.4 |
| *Weakened social control* | | | | |
| Normlessness | 0.5 | 0.4 | 0.3 | 0.5 |
| Live alone (%) | 1.6 | 1.5 | 3 | 21.3 |
| *Sample size* | 1,100 | 2,176 | 183 | 484 |

Results are based on 'svytab' and 'svymean' analysis in STATA and adjusted for sampling probability and survey design

For sexual risk of HIV, data in Table 16.2 reveal that non-*hukou* migrants had a significantly higher likelihood of having had sex with a casual partner in the 30 days prior to the survey than any of the other three migrant/non-migrant groups. However, the likelihood of having unprotected casual sex did not vary significantly across the migrant and non-migrant groups, although non-*hukou* migrants did show the highest percentage. In terms of the overall sexual risk of HIV, as measured by the composite index, non-*hukou* migrants again were at highest risk. In all three measures, no statistical significance was found between *hukou* migrants and non-migrants or between the two non-migrant groups. For more definitive analyses, we now turn to multiple regression analysis.

When only migrant status variables are included, the results in Table 16.3 mirror those in Table 16.2 but in odds ratio format. Being a non-*hukou* migrant was associated with significantly higher odds of having sex with casual partner(s) in the month prior to interview (Model 1). However, migrant and non-migrant groups did not differ significantly in the odds of having unprotected casual sex (Model 3). In other words, while non-*hukou* migrants were more likely to have casual sex, they were about equal in the likelihood of using condoms in casual sex.

The control of individual demographic characteristics and measures of social isolation/social control (Model 2) reduced considerably the odds ratio between non-*hukou* migrant and rural non-migrant (from 7.5 to 5.5 or 27 per cent reduction) for having casual sex, indicating that on average non-*hukou* migrants' demographic characteristics and psychosocial well-being, measured by social isolation/social control, were conducive to having casual sex. However, even after demographic characteristics and psychosocial well-being were controlled for, non-*hukou* migrants remained more than five times as likely as comparable rural non-migrants to have had casual sex in the month prior to the interview.

None of the four demographic characteristics showed any significant association with the odds of having casual sex (Model 2). But being male was associated with significantly higher odds (more than double) of having unprotected casual sex (Model 4). Among measures of social isolation and control, depression was

*Table 16.2* HIV risk sexual behaviours in the 30 days prior to interview, by migrant status

| HIV risk sexual behaviour | Rural non-migrants | Urban non-migrants | Hukou migrants | Non-hukou migrants |
|---|---|---|---|---|
| Having casual sex (%) | 2.4* | 4.0* | 1.8* | 15.6 |
| Having unprotected casual sex (%) | 1.7 | 2.4 | 1.7 | 2.8 |
| Sexual risk of HIV Index (mean) | 0.2* | 0.2* | 0.1* | 0.6 |
| *Sample size* | 1,071 | 2,111 | 172 | 470 |

Results are based on 'svytab' and 'svymean' analysis in STATA and adjusted for sampling probability and survey design. Statistical significance tests are based on comparison to non-*hukou* rural–urban migrants
*$p<0.01$

*Table 16.3* Multiple logistic regression analysis of the odds of having casual and unprotected casual sex with non-regular partner(s) in the 30 days prior to the interview[a]

| Independentvariables[b] | Casual sex | | Unprotected casual sex | |
|---|---|---|---|---|
| | Model 1 | Model 2 | Model 3 | Model 4 |
| *Migrant status* | | | | |
| Urban non-migrant | 1.713 | 1.753 | 1.458 | 1.474 |
| Rural–urban *hukou* migrant | 0.752 | 0.761 | 1.032 | 1.309 |
| Rural–urban non-*hukou* migrant | 7.538** | 5.481** | 1.683 | 1.81 |
| *Demographic characteristics* | | | | |
| Age | | 0.998 | | 0.996 |
| Male | | 1.421 | | 2.759* |
| Married | | 0.537 | | 0.981 |
| Education[c] | | 0.892 | | 1.026 |
| *Social isolation* | | | | |
| Economic marginalization | | 0.962 | | 1.007 |
| Loneliness | | 0.995 | | 0.988 |
| Depression | | 1.095** | | 1.120** |
| *Weakened social control* | | | | |
| Live alone | | 1.287 | | 0.169** |
| Normlessness | | 1.486** | | 1.157 |
| *Model F* | 8.37** | 18.31** | 0.19 | 12.06** |
| *Sample size* | 3,824 | 3,791 | 3,824 | 3,791 |

[a] Results are maximum likelihood estimates based on the 'svylogit' model for dichotomous dependent variable in STATA software and expressed as the odds ratios, adjusted for sampling probability and survey design
[b] The reference categories for variables of migrant status, male, married, and live alone are rural non-migrant, female, single, and live with others, respectively
[c] Education is entered as an ordinal variable: 1 illiterate or semi-illiterate; 2 elementary school; 3 junior high school; 4 senior high school; 5 vocational school; 6 two/three years college; and 7 four years college or more
$*p<0.05$; $**p<0.01$

significantly associated with odds of having unprotected casual sex. The normlessness index remained significantly associated with the odds of having casual sex (Model 2) but was not statistically significant for the odds of having unprotected casual sex (Model 4). Perhaps surprisingly, Model 4 suggests that living alone was significantly associated with a much lower likelihood of having unprotected casual sex (OR = 0.17).

When the composite index measuring the overall sexual risk of HIV is examined, the linear regression analysis results in Table 16.4 suggested being a non-*hukou* migrant was significantly and positively associated with the composite index. The control of demographic characteristics and measures of social isolation/social control made little difference. The result suggested that in terms of overall risk, as measured by the composite index, non-*hukou* migrants were on average at significantly greater sexual risk of HIV than *hukou* migrants and/or non-migrants. It appears that even though non-*hukou* migrants might have a similar rate (probability) of condom use in casual sex than *hukou* migrants or non-migrants (Table 16.3, Model 4), as captured by the composite index, they had

*Table 16.4* Multiple linear regression analysis of overall sexual risk of HIV in the 30 days prior to the interview[a]

| | Overall sexual risk of HIV | |
|---|---|---|
| Independent variables[b] | Model 1 | Model 2 |
| *Migrant status* | | |
| Urban non-migrant | 0.057 | 0.093 |
| Rural–urban *hukou* migrant | −0.057 | 0.003 |
| Rural–urban non-*hukou* migrant | 0.412* | 0.348* |
| *Demographic characteristics* | | |
| Age | | <0.001 |
| Male | | 0.126* |
| Married | | −0.009 |
| Education[c] | | −0.032 |
| *Social isolation* | | |
| Economic marginalization | | −0.001 |
| Loneliness | | −0.001 |
| Depression | | 0.013* |
| *Weakened social control* | | |
| Live alone | | 0.194 |
| Normlessness | | 0.177* |
| *Model F* | 9.07* | 12.50* |
| *Sample size* | 3,943 | 3,910 |

[a] Results are the coefficient estimates based on the 'svyreg' model for continuous dependent variable in STATA software, adjusted for sampling probability and survey design
[b] The reference categories for variables of migrant status, male, married, and live alone are rural non-migrant, female, single, and live with others, respectively
[c] Education is entered as an ordinal variable: 1 illiterate or semi-illiterate; 2 elementary school; 3 junior high school; 4 senior high school; 5 vocational school; 6 two/three years college; and 7 four years college or more
* $p < 0.01$

more unprotected casual sex because of their greater numbers of casual sexual partners and casual sexual acts and/or had riskier casual sexual partners, such as commercial sex workers and injection drug users. Among the control variables, being male was significantly and positively associated with the composite sexual risk index, as were extent of depression and experiences of normlessness.

Interestingly however, and consistent with prior research (Yang and Xia 2008), the analysis also found that differences in risk behaviours of migrants and non-migrants were more pronounced amongst females than males, suggesting that the nature and effects of migration are gender influenced.[1]

## Conclusions

Within two decades, HIV and AIDS have evolved from perceived diseases of foreigners to an expanding epidemic affecting every population group in China. Using data from a population-based survey that included both migrants and non-migrants, the analysis here has focused on the impact of rural–urban non-*hukou* migration on the likelihood of having casual and/or unprotected sex as well as the overall sexual risk of HIV.

The results suggest that rural–urban non-*hukou* migrants in China are indeed more likely than both *hukou* migrants and non-migrants to have sex with casual partners. Rural–urban *hukou* migrants, by contrast, are no more likely than comparable non-migrants to have casual sex. Although rural–urban non-*hukou* migrants' increased casual sex does not appear to be associated with the measure of unprotected casual sex, overall sexual risk of HIV as measured by the analysis' composite index is also significantly higher among rural–urban non-*hukou* migrants.

To some extent, the selectivity of rural–urban non-*hukou* migrants by age (high concentration aged 18–29) and marital status (higher proportion unmarried) may contribute to their increased sexual risk of HIV. But the lack of a local permanent *hukou* is likely the key to rural–urban non-*hukou* migrants' increased risk of HIV. In the unique Chinese context, the lack of a local permanent *hukou* in the city hinders or prevents post-migration integration and consequently increases a non-*hukou* migrant's social isolation in the urban destination. For all measures of social isolation/social control, non-*hukou* migrants on average fared worse than *hukou* migrants or non-migrants, and both social isolation and social control were found to be significantly associated with casual sex and the overall sexual risk of HIV.

However, even after measures of social isolation/social control were controlled for, rural–urban non-*hukou* migrants remain most likely to have casual sex and to be at the highest overall sexual risk of HIV. This suggests that factors other than social isolation and weakened social control are also contributing to non-*hukou* migrants' increased sexual risk of HIV. Future research is needed to identify these factors and to better understand the mechanisms that link rural–urban non-*hukou* migration to sexual risk of HIV. Until then, it is important for policy makers in China to consider reforming the *hukou* system to allow rural–urban non-*hukou* migrants to register in the system and to de-link access to all government employment and social services from the possession of a local permanent *hukou*. The integration of non-*hukou* migrants into the system and the removal of the divide between local *hukou* haves and have-nots would facilitate the full integration of rural–urban non-*hukou* migrants in cities, reduce their social isolation, and increase their social attachment and bonding to mainstream urban societies.

## Notes

1 Data are not presented here but are available upon request.

## References

Anderson, A., Qingsi, Z., Hua, X., and Jianfeng, B. (2003) 'China's floating population and the potential for HIV transmission: A social-behavioural perspective', *AIDS Care*, 152: 177–85.

Bilsborrow, R. E., Hugo, G. J., Oberai, A. S., and Zlotnik, H. (1997) *International Migration Statistics: Guidelines for the Improvement of Data Collection Systems*, Geneva: International Labour Office.

Black, D. (1984) *Toward a General Theory of Social Control*, New York: Academic Press, Inc.

Cheng, T. and Selden, M. (1994) 'The origins and social consequences of China's Hukou system', *The China Quarterly*, 139: 644–68.

Coser, L. A. (1982) 'The notion of control in sociological theory', in J. P. Gibbs (ed.), *Social Control: Views from the Social Sciences*, Beverly Hills, California: Sage Publications, Inc., pp. 13–22.

Emler, N. (1999) 'Moral character', in V. Derlega, B. Winstead, and W. Jones (eds), *Personality: Contemporary Theory and Research*, Chicago, Illinois: Nelson-Hall, pp. 376–404.

Fan, C. (2002) 'The elite, the natives, and the outsiders: Migration and labor market segmentation in urban China', *Annals of the Association of American Geographers*, 92(1): 103–24.

Farrer, J. (2002) *Opening Up: Youth Sex Culture and Market Reform in Shanghai*, Chicago, Illinois: The University of Chicago Press.

Gibbs, J. P. (1982) *Social Control: Views from the Social Sciences*, Beverly Hills, California: Sage Publications, Inc.

Hu, Z., Liu, H., Li, X., Stanton, B., and Chen, X. (2006) 'HIV-related sexual behaviour among migrants and non-migrants in a rural area of China: Role of rural-to-urban migration', *Public Health*, 120: 339–45.

Knight, J., Song, L., and Jia, H. (1999) 'Chinese rural migrants in urban enterprises: Three perspectives', *Journal of Development Studies*, 35(3): 73–104.

Li, Xiaoming, Zhang, Liying, Stanton, Bonita, Fang, Xiaoyi, Xiong, Qing, and Lin, Danhua (2007) 'HIV/AIDS-related sexual risk behaviours among rural residents in China: Potential role of rural-to-urban migration', *AIDS Education and Prevention*, 19(5): 396–407.

Liang, Z. and Ma, Z. (2004) 'China's floating population: New evidence from the 2000 Census', *Population and Development Review*, 30: 467–88.

Ma, L. and Xiang, B. (1998) 'Native place, migration and the emergence of peasant enclaves in Beijing', *The China Quarterly*, 155: 546–81.

Merli, M. Giovanna, Hertog, Sara, Wang, Bo, and Li, Jing (2006) 'Modelling the spread of HIV/AIDS in China: The role of sexual transmission', *Population Studies*, 60 (1): 1–22.

NBS (National Bureau of Statistics of China) (2008) *Communiqué on Major Data of the Second National Agricultural Census of China (no. 5)*, Beijing: NBS.

Pan, S. W. Parish, A. Wang, and E. Laumann (2004) *Sexual Behaviours and Sexual Relationships in Contemporary China*, Beijing: Social Science Manuscripts Publisher.

Parish, W. L., E. O. Laumann, M. S. Cohen, S. Pan, H. Zheng, I. Hoffman, T. Wang, and K. H. Ng (2003) 'Population-based study of Chlamydial infection in China', *Journal of American Medical Association*, 289(10): 1265–73.

Radloff, L. S. (1977) 'The CES-D Scale: A self-report depression scale for research in the general population', *Applied Psychological Measurement*, 1: 385–401.

Roberts, K. (1997) 'China's "tidal wave" of migrant labor: What can we learn from Mexican undocumented migration to the United States?', *International Migration Review*, 31: 249–93.

Russell, D. W. (1996) 'UCLA Loneliness Scale (Version 3): Reliability, validity, and factor structure', *Journal of Personality Assessment*, 66: 20–40.

Smith, C. J. and Yang, X. (2005) 'Examining the connection between temporary migration and the spread of STIs and HIV/AIDS in China', *The China Review*, 5: 109–37.

Solinger, D. (1999) *Contesting Citizenship in Urban China: Peasant Migrants, the State, and the Logic of the Market*, Berkeley, California: University of California.

State Council AIDS Working Committee Office and the United Nations Theme Group on AIDS (2008) *UNGASS Country Progress Report: P. R. China*, New York: UNAIDS.

Troyer, R., Clark, J., and Rojek, D. (1989) *Social Control in the People's Republic of China*, New York: Praeger.

van den Hoek, A., Yuliang, F., Dukers, N. H., Zhiheng, C., Jiangting, F., Lina, Z., and Xiuxing, Z. (2001) 'High prevalence of Syphilis and other sexually transmitted diseases among sex workers in China: Potential for fast spread of HIV', *AIDS*, 15: 753–59.

Wang, F. L. (2004) 'Reformed migration control and new targeted people: China's hukou system in the 2000s', *The China Quarterly*, 177: 115–32.

Wang, F., Zuo, X., and Ruan, D. (2002) 'Rural migrants in Shanghai: Living under the shadow of socialism', *International Migration Review*, 36(2): 520–645.

Whyte, M. and Parish, W. (1984) *Urban Life in Contemporary China*, Chicago, Illinois: University of Chicago Press.

Williams, M., McCoy, H. V., Brown, A., Saunders, L., Freeman, R., and Chen, D. (2001) 'An evaluation of a brief HIV risk reduction intervention using empirically derived drug use and sexual risk indices', *AIDS and Behavior*, 5: 31–43.

Wilson, W. J. (1987) *The Truly Disadvantaged: The Inner City, the Underclass, and Public Policy*, Chicago, Illinois: University of Chicago Press.

Yan, Y. (2003) *Private Life Under Socialism: Love, Intimacy, and Family Change in a Chinese Village, 1949–1999*, Stanford, California: Stanford University Press.

Yang, X. (1993) 'Household registration, economic reform, and migration', *International Migration Review*, 27(4): 796–818.

—— (2006) 'Temporary migration and HIV risk behaviors in China', *Environment and Planning A*, 38: 1527–43.

Yang, X., Derlega, V., and Luo, H. (2007) 'Migration, behaviour change, and HIV/STD risks in China', *AIDS Care*, 19: 282–88.

Yang, X. and Xia, G. (2008) 'Temporary migration and STD/HIV risky sexual behavior: A population-based analysis of gender differences in China', *Social Problems*, 55(3): 322–46.

Zhang, K., Li, D., Li, H., and Beck, E. J. (1999) 'Changing sexual attitudes and behaviour in China: Implications for the spread of HIV and other sexually transmitted diseases', *AIDS Care*, 11(5): 581–89.

Zhang, L. (2001) *Strangers in the City: Reconfigurations of Space, Power, and Social Networks within China's Floating Population*, Stanford, California: Stanford University Press.

# Index